Praise for *Shoot My Ashes from a Cannon* by Danni Fourton Morford

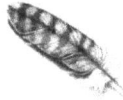

"In *Shoot My Ashes from a Cannon,* Danni Morford reminds us that the best path forward in life is unflinching honesty. The best companions for this journey are humor and faith. And the greatest gift is the transcendent love of family."
—Andrew Wainwright, Author:
It's Not Okay to Be a Cannibal: How to Keep Addiction from Eating Your Family Alive

"There are lessons throughout, not just of the utter tragedy of addiction but also the uplifting possibility and downright necessity of recovery for those who are left behind after the illness moves on."
—William C. Moyers
New York Times Best-Selling Author

""Exquisitely painful and achingly gorgeous, Danni's collection of letters is a true gift."
—Sandy Swenson, Author:
The Joey Song & Tending Dandelions

i

"Danni's no shame approach to facing adversity with truth and humor is refreshing and powerful. *Shoot My Ashes* is emotional and insightful. This is a valuable book for anyone struggling in the realm of addiction."

—Lisa Bovee
Author and Founder of *Guided by Grief*

SHOOT MY ASHES
FROM A CANNON

SHOOT MY ASHES FROM A CANNON

FROM A CANNON

Beyond Addiction

The Letters

Danni Fourton Morford

MOON
DOG
M.L.P.

Dedications

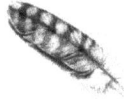

TRAVIS, our brown-eyed boy, a loving son, brother and friend. Gone too soon, but will never, ever be forgotten.

Pete, my husband of 45 years who has traveled this journey with me. Thank you for your support and help with my book, for nourishing me with your delicious cooking; holding me when I was exhausted. Thank you for being a loving husband, nurturing father and my best friend.

Eric, thank you for showing me that it is never too late to go after your dreams. Your bike sojourn and your walk on The Pacific Coast Trail were an inspiration for me to walk the Camino de Santiago. Thank you for being strong in your faith and your love of family. For never giving up and for meeting life head on. You continue to amaze me.

Caleb, you made hard choices early in life for which you are now reaping the benefits of a happy and healthy life style. Thank you for being my trainer for years and keeping me strong. You have a calm and easy-going spirit. Your caring and compassionate nature is a tremendous support to our family. I continue to learn from you on a daily basis.

Ashley, you are the daughter I never had, and such a beautiful blessing. You continue to embrace our crazy family and enrich our lives. Your passion for good health and the desire to share your lifestyle is to be admired. Thank you for loving us and being Caleb's soul mate.

Contents

Foreword

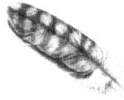

RARELY DO I endorse or offer my support on behalf of other people's literary endeavors. My own writing keeps me creatively focused and by opening the door even slightly I invite a rush of people who want my support. I simply don't have the time much less the energy, except in rare instances.

Danni Morford's project is one of these rare instances. She knows firsthand the power of addiction. For years, she and her family wrestled with the insidious beast that grabbed and wouldn't let go of a son until the day he succumbed to this chronic illness. Their loss is complete. But it isn't the end of their story.

Danni has turned the adversity of her family's tragedy into the opportunity to help others by way of what is perhaps a unique storytelling genre: the family's annual Christmas letter.

Through these holiday letters (and others that she writes after her son died), Danni shares insights and emotions that are unique to her experience as a mother living with and experiencing the death of a child due to addiction.

Yet sadly, what happened to her family is not unique; millions of people know first-hand the power of addiction and what too often happens before and after to families of loved ones who cannot recover. That's what makes Danni Morford's book worth reading. There are lessons throughout, not just of the utter tragedy of addiction but also the uplifting possibility and downright necessity of recovery for those who are left behind after the illness moves on.

Danni has been on both sides of the experience, and her uncanny ability to intimately share her journey through the spirit of holiday letters to family and friends, makes all of us her fellow travelers. Despite her loss, it is hope that her book is all about. I urge you to read it, and you'll agree.

—William C. Moyers
New York Times Best-Selling Author
Broken: My Story of Addiction and Redemption
Vice President of Public Affairs & Community Relations
Hazelden Betty Ford Foundation

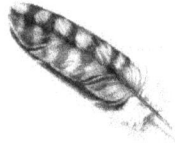

"I truly believe God has a greater plan for us, and we can't fulfill it if we are strung out, dead, or incarcerated, so don't get down on yourself and realize this too shall pass."

~ **Travis Morford**

Origins of The Christmas Letter

—

2019

At first, my Christmas Letter was an outlet to use humor and to be truthful about my family. I was tired of reading such BS in Christmas letters that came in the mail every year, and I knew most of my friends, especially my Al-Anon® friends, felt the same way. Maybe I was jealous, but other letters left me feeling like a bad parent – like I'd somehow screwed up along the way.

By writing these letters, I could spill my guts and figure out what was going on with me emotionally, so I'm grateful my family gave the thumbs-up to send them. This is a story of my family and the power of letters. Over the years they've helped me realize my family has just the right amount of crazy mixed with a whole lot of love. I hope my letters will bring about awareness to the Disease of Addiction.

Blessings,
Danni

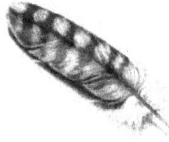

"While we try and teach our children all about life, our children teach us what life is all about."
~ **Angela Schwindt**

The Letters

The Christmas Letter

—

2004

Dear Friends,

It's been a busy year. The boys are all doing various activities. Unfortunately, most of it is illegal.

They did graduate from the Shoal Creek Intensive Outpatient Program. It seemed like they'd received a "bachelor's degree" in drug management. We are sincerely hoping they don't go for their master's degree.

Eric "starred" in a video that was filmed in Mexico while he was on Spring break. It was a video shot and directed by the police. You guessed it: Eric was taking the field-test for sobriety. After starring in the video, he was awarded a ten-day vacation at the jail in Brownsville, Texas. The accommodations weren't very nice, the food sucked, and it was crowded. He had to share a room with twelve other people, none of whom spoke English.

One day in November, Caleb called to tell me he'd been driving drunk and ran into someone's yard, but not to worry because he called the police on himself. Boy, was I proud!

Caleb told the officer that he was tired of struggling with his addiction and wanted to go to treatment. He was not arrested, but he was given a ticket. The next day, the policeman came to our house and said that he'd never had anything like this happen before. He tore the ticket up because he thought Caleb would make the right choice. After this happened Caleb asked to go to treatment, which was a first for us. On Thanksgiving Day, we took a family trip and took him to Camp Recovery where he stayed for 6 months.

As you can tell, our family is big on traditions, and the boys try hard to keep them going. They never let a holiday go by without a call from jail or someone in detox. Bless their sweet hearts, you've got to love them.

I was thinking the other day what it would be like to write a country song about my family. It would probably go something like this:

> My dog can't play with the
> neighbor's dog 'cause he bit him on
> the head.
> My son can't drive down the street,
> cause that's what the neighbors said.
> A visit from the DEA, a policeman
> now and then.
> Oh Lord my prayers were answered
> when you gave me three young sons.
> I should have prayed for clean and
> sober ones.

Anyway, you get the idea. I am really happy to tell you that I finally got an Al-Anon® sponsor. It is great! I can talk with her for hours and the best part...IT'S FREE!

Well, I need to go now – looks like a police cruiser just pulled in the drive. I hope I managed to spread a little cheer.

Merry Christmas from the Morfords; we will be back again next year.

Love,

Danni

The Christmas Letter

—

2005

Dear Friends,

Merry Christmas from the Morfords – the family that knows how to put the fun into dysFUNctional. This year consisted of three active boys, two dogs, a workaholic spouse and me wearing a scarlet "C" for trying to control.

Pete and I celebrated our 31st anniversary. We hardly ever fight anymore; I just detach and leave. Pete is currently commuting to the Woodlands and plans to retire in June.

Caleb finished his six months of treatment and graduated in May. He received his one-year AA birthday chip this November. We are so very proud of him.

Eric finished out his probation. He graduated from The Short Program, with only two tickets and a little fender bender, so things are looking up for him.

Travis found his soul mate; they have a lot in common. Both are trust fund babies; thanks to my dear sweet monster-in-law... I mean mother-in-law. They also share a love for the same drugs and excitement only addicts can experience. We also found out she was pregnant. Unfortunately, she miscarried when she was in jail. I think the stress of the Swat Team arresting her was just too much.

On the bright side, we conducted an intervention for Travis, and he went to treatment. So, our family was able to go to two more family weekends, which are always so much fun. To be in a roomful of other families in crisis is so uplifting, you can just feel the love.

I must confess, I had a few relapses myself this year. I enabled my kids a time or two and gave unsolicited advice often. I even repeated it several times, just in case they didn't hear me. My new motto is, "a meeting a day, keeps my addicts at bay."

I continue to go to meetings and enjoy connecting with my "Step Sisters." It is nice to have friends who can understand, listen, and relate to me.

I can't believe another year has come and gone. God has truly blessed us. I am thankful for all the trials and the lessons learned. It is comforting to know when I step out of the way, God can and does work miracles.

As always, I hope I was able to spread a little cheer.

Merry Christmas from the Morfords; we will be back again next year.

Love,

Danni

The Christmas Letter

—

2006

Dear Friends,

Hope y'all are doing well. We sure had a great year; Travis finished up treatment in Louisiana and has been working and living in a sober house. In October, he was ordered by the State of Texas to return home and begin probation. As a welcome home gift, The Court presented him with a cute gadget called an Interlock Breathalyzer Device (IBD) for his truck. It is very easy to work, especially if you don't drink alcohol.

Last year, he damaged a neighbor's tree while driving under the influence. I am happy to say the tree is flourishing thanks in part to Travis's dog, Tyson kept it fertilized while on our daily walks.

On a positive note Travis is taking courses to get certified as a personal trainer, and he is also doing some landscape work.

Eric managed to go on a trip this year, unfortunately it was a trip on acid. The police were called, and he was arrested. Pete was out of town and missed all the excitement. After the "trip," Eric went to treatment, and he managed to last a month before he was asked to leave – he was not working the program.

Once again, all my boys are back in Texas; guess this is where they are meant to be. Eric's time in jail made an impression on him. He started making better choices and took a very strong interest in his health and well-being through diet, exercise, and avoidance of drugs and alcohol.

Caleb is doing well; he got a job and moved to his own apartment, he pays his rent, and has a darling girlfriend. I was informed that she was upset because I never mention her in my Christmas letters. I tried explaining she really did not want to be in them and to be careful what she wished for.

We had a small window of opportunity when all the boys were doing really well; we were able to take a family vacation to Europe for 3 weeks. It was a great trip and one I will look back on with fond memories. The boys had so much fun and Pete and I loved showing them Europe for the first time. Travis even pointed out to me the AA symbol of a meetinghouse in Prague. I don't mean to brag, but our family could almost pass for normal.

So, Dear Friends, I hope we were able to spread some Christmas cheer. Merry Christmas from the Morfords.

We will be back again next year.

Love,

Danni

The Christmas Letter

—

2007

Dear Friends,

I wondered if I would be able to write to you this year. It is the hardest letter I have ever had to write, but I knew it was important to do so. I wish I could say it has been an uneventful year, but then I would be lying, and this is all about The True Christmas Letter.

I want you to know that Travis died on July 8th from an overdose of hydrocodone, Xanax, and alcohol. He was 25 years old. He fought hard, but the disease of addiction proved to be too strong for him. Our family is not ashamed to say Travis died from addiction. In telling Travis's story, we hope that others will learn about the disease of addiction and lives can be saved.

On the day of Travis's memorial service, my brother Happy died from a heart attack; he was trying to get home for the funeral.

Happy had been in Alaska on a cruise; he was 57 years old. There were days when I didn't think I could make it or if our family would survive the loss of Travis, which was most certainly compounded by the death of my brother.

It has been five months since Travis died; our family is learning a new normal. Grief has been our teacher. God, family, and the love of our friends have meant so much to us.

Travis may be gone, but he will never be forgotten; he will live forever in our hearts.

So Dear Friends, please know that our family is even closer in our time of grief. Peace be with you always. Hope and Faith.

Merry Christmas from The Morfords.

We will be back again next year.

Love,

Danni

My Closet

—

2007

Dear Travis,

I wanted to find a way that I could still talk to you. Communicating through a letter or a note still seems the most comfortable way. There are times when I need a place to go and sit and be alone with my thoughts. It seems like I always end up in my closet sitting on the floor hidden by my clothes. Your sweet dog, Tyson, found this place too, so we share this hideaway. I have a soft blanket for him to lie on.

My chair is the floor and I lean against the wall and just think, feel, and breathe. I think that your dad thinks I'm weird, but he is getting used to the new me.

Our new normal...It sucks.

Love you brown-eyed boy,

Mom

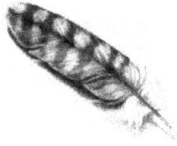

"More than kisses, letters mingle souls."
~ John Donne

The Obituary

—

2007

Dear Travis,

I had to write your obituary today, which is something no parent should ever have to do. Your dad had been in Singapore for two months, and he is trying to get home. I had to call and tell him the horrible news; I could feel his grief from across the ocean.

Your friend Connor was at the house and he sat down to help me with it. I asked Connor to write that you died from the F.........g disease of addiction. He looked at me with compassion and said, "Danni, I don't think you can say that in the paper." I said, "I know Connor, but I just need to see the words written."

Travis, I will always remember when you told me how you hated being an addict and how at times you would ask God to let you die. To hear you say those words broke my heart. You were a fighter and fought this disease from a young age.

I promise we will do everything we can to bring awareness to this disease. In sharing our family's story, our hope is that others will share their stories too and help rid addiction of the stigma that makes it hard to ask for help and to recover.

Love you, Mom

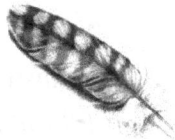

"Being a mother is learning about strengths you
didn't know you had and dealing with fear you
didn't know existed."

~ Linda Wooten

Beloved Dog of Travis

—

2007

Dear Travis,

I remember when you first brought Tyson to meet us. He was the cutest little puppy I had ever seen. He was like your shadow and followed you everywhere. His face holds so much expression, especially in his eyes. I asked you why you wanted a pit bull and you answered that you wanted people to know they are good, loyal dogs. I am happy you chose him.

He has given us so much joy and become a part of our family. Tyson is my walking buddy. We take long walks at Town lake and in the neighborhood. I began to realize he faced the same judgment and stigma an addict faces each day. Just like people have no idea about this breed of dog, people have no idea about this horrible disease of addiction. I am sorry that you had such a hard battle with a disease where so much stigma and shame are attached. I say your name often and tell Tyson how much you loved him.

Love you,

Mom

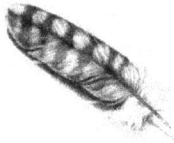

"No more shame. No more silence."
~ **Sandy Swenson**

Message in a Bottle

—

July 2007

Dear Travis,

I had to write to you this night. It has only been a few weeks since you died. The family decided to keep the plans of going to Port Aransas. We hope to find some peace away from home. To be honest, it is so very hard to be at this place – the memories keep flooding in.

The waves you loved to chase now hit us full force and try to knock us down. There is no rhythm to our pain. I wonder if we will survive life without you.

We found some bottles and wrote messages to you and sealed them up. Later, when it was dark, we walked in silence down the beach to the jetties, and we tossed the bottles in the ocean. We sat there in the quietness where stillness lives and felt the moonbeams pull at our heartstrings.

Your footprints left their mark upon our hearts.

Love you always,

Mom

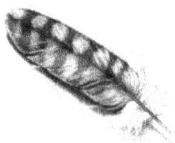

"Give sorrow words."
~ **William Shakespeare**

The Gift of Letters

—

2007

Dear Travis,

Several weeks after you died, the letters started arriving in the mail from your friends and ours. They thought we would like to have the letters you had written to them. We were very touched by their thoughtfulness.

Your letters and familiar handwriting were comforting to me, as was the tangible feel of the paper. This visual of you taking the time to write and the effort of your deep reflection, told me how much you cared for the person receiving your letter.

Your handwriting revealed the struggle it took for you to write at times when you were deep in your addiction. The depth and intimacy of your words are powerful. What you wrote to comfort others is now comforting me. Thank you for this gift of letters.

Your letters will live on and become your legacy.

Love you darling son,

Mom

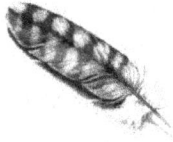

"Letters are among the most significant memorial
a person can leave behind."
~ Johann Wolfgang von Goethe

Bringing Him Home

—

2007

Dear Travis,

One day in August of 2007, I received a phone call to inform me that your ashes were ready. I was grateful no one was home to go with me; this was something I wanted to do by myself. Driving there that day, I felt like I was in a haze of nothingness and moving in slow motion. I am thinking 'how can this be happening?'

I arrived at the funeral home, entered and encountered a sickening smell of flowers; a smell that will always remind me of your death. Flowers that once brought me joy, now bring me sorrow. I followed the funeral director, Kenneth, down a dimly lit hallway, the whole atmosphere was one of suffocating silence. He asked me to take a seat in his office and wait; my heart and soul were sick; the finality of all that had happened was coming to the surface once again.

Kenneth returned carrying a velvet bag. I thanked him as he handed me your ashes. I took your ashes, held you close and walked out the door. I opened the front passenger door of the car and gently set you on the seat, it was good to be taking you home.

Where do you go when you can't go any further? The spirit must endure, and you continue down the road the extra mile.

You trust.

Love you forever,

Mom

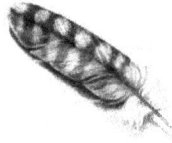

"Write hard and clear about what hurts."

~ **Ernest Hemingway**

The Shrine

—

August 2007

Dear Travis,

We have a shrine on the wall by our bed where your ashes are kept along with blue jay feathers and a picture of you. As a child, you were afraid of the dark. I wanted you near me and dad. Before I go to bed, I kiss you and tell you that we love you. Some of your friends asked if they could have some of your ashes, I said yes because I felt that would be alright with you.

The times when I have your ashes feels so holy. To hold you in my hands, knowing that this will be the only way I will ever get to be close to you. This experience causes me to reach another depth of sadness I didn't know I could feel. When I am left with your ashes on my hands, I cannot wash you off. I just can't wash you down the drain. So, I rub your ashes into my neck and chest and across my heart. I breathe you in then lick the ashes off, and you become a part of me again.

Always loving you,

Mom

27

"Sometimes sighing is the only way I can breathe."

~ Danni Morford

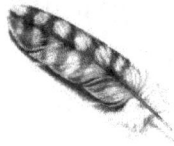

The Coroner's Report

—

September 2007

Dear Travis,

We received the Medical Examiner's report today. I did not want to read the letter but felt it was something I needed to do. The report stated you were a young healthy male: your heart, lungs, and nervous system were all normal. It went on in great detail and listed the tattoos you had and any small scars. The Death Certificate indicated your death from an "accidental overdose from a mixture of Alprazolam, Hydrocodone, marijuana, alcohol & antihistamines."

You had taken so many drugs that your lungs were congested, and you could not breathe. I wonder if there will ever be a time when a Death Certificate states someone died from the Disease of Addiction.

Travis, when you stopped by the house that afternoon, you looked great and seemed so happy. You were excited about starting your job as a personal trainer.

When you left, you gave me a big hug and kiss. I didn't know this would be the last time I would ever see you again. It has only been a few weeks now, since you've been gone, but at times it feels like you have been gone for years.

29

Travis you are free now. I am grateful you have no more pain from this disease. You fought a valiant fight, and you will always be my hero.

Forever loving you,

Mom

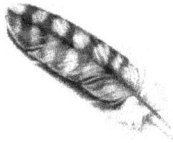

"Grief is the courage to feel the loss, even though
you feel you can no longer stand it."
~ *One Day at a Time in Al-Anon*

The Christi Center

—

2007

Dear Travis,

On a cold November night of 2007, I attended my first grief support meeting. The meeting took place in an old Central Austin neighborhood off 45th street. A modest gray home sits with a Purple Heart sign that reads: "The Christi Center." I had driven past the house so many times over the years, never knowing its history or function.

Susan and Don lost their daughter, Christi, who was hit by a drunk driver in 1981. Susan is the founder of this place originally named "The Love of Christi." Susan greeted me at the door that night. She is a petite woman in her 60s with warm sparkling brown eyes. A sense of peace radiated from her. It was easy talking with her, as she asked questions about you and our family and shared with me about her daughter. Susan took me to the room where the other moms meet each Monday night.

The room I entered was warm and cozy. The walls were painted a delicate lilac, where paintings were hung with angels and hearts. There were comfortable chairs and couches where 20 or so women gathered. This group I joined was one no one ever wants to be a part of: a group of moms who had lost a child. The room was filled with broken hearts and shattered dreams and moms in different stages of grief.

As I sat there and listened to their stories, I looked at the faces around me. These beautiful moms had eyes that were liquid pools of sorrow and deep lines were etched upon their faces. Some were so tightly wound you could feel the tension in their necks. They talked the language of grief, a deep sigh, and the question why? They spoke confessions of regret. For two very long hours we talked and cried, sharing what we were going through. During this meeting, Susan shared with us that there is no word in the English dictionary for a parent whose child has died. I feel this is because no name or word could ever adequately describe this devastating loss.

At the close of the meeting, Susan spoke for a few more minutes and reassured us that our feelings and emotions were "normal," and we weren't going crazy.

I left feeling so very drained. Listening to so many stories of grief was difficult.

I wondered if I would be able to sleep.

Missing you,

Love,

Mom

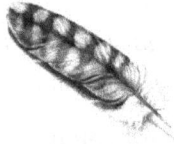

"Sometimes our light goes out but is blown into flame by another human being. Each of us owes deepest thanks to those who have rekindled this light."

~ **Albert Schweitzer**

Midnight Baby

—

November 2007

Dear Travis,

I woke up this morning with you on my mind. I just laid there and thought of you. Your sweet dog, Tyson, curled up next to me. I think he senses that I am sad and tries to comfort me with doggy kisses. Do you remember when I sang lullabies to you, when we rocked away to never-land? Your tiny fingers curled around a lock of my hair as you gazed up at me with your brown eyes; you were my midnight baby.

You are in the air I breathe; you are in the shooting stars, you are in the night moon, and the blue jay's feather. All of these are sweet moments; you are never far from me. Your dad and brothers miss you too. I can see it in their eyes and hear it in their voices.

Grief surrounds us, and though no one says it, we know our family will never be the same. It hurts. I cannot wait till that mother/child reunion.

Until then, I will carry you forever in my heart.

Always loving you,

Mom

"You stole my heart.
You were the sweetest baby I had ever seen.
You were my Midnight Baby."
~ **Danni Morford**

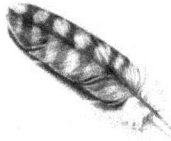

The Christmas Eve Letter

—

2007

Dear Travis,

The first Christmas Eve without you was very hard. I could not sleep, so I went and sat in the den and listened to the song, "Oh Holy Night." Hearing the words of joy and hope calmed me, allowing my emotions to unwrap the memories of Christmas past.

I started a new tradition of writing a letter to you which, when complete, I place in your Christmas stocking.

I write about Tyson, your brothers, your dad, and how proud you would be of them.

Merry Christmas darling.

I love you,

Mom

DANNI MORFORD

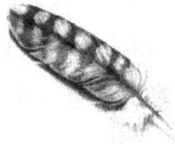

"This holiest of nights, I picture you in heaven surrounded by the sound of angels singing."
~ **Henry Wadsworth Longfellow**

The Christmas Letter

—

2008

Dear Friends,

This has been a year of "Firsts:" Travis's birthday, his first "Angel Date," and all the other first days and holidays that have come and gone without him here with us.

This has also been a year of observing how each one of us has dealt with our grief. Pete has always been a workaholic and with grief these days it's like he is on steroids. Why, it wears me out to just watch him! He is an engineer and tries to fix me and sometimes I can't be fixed. Being "the good wife," I told him he was not grieving the right way, which he did not want to hear.

Eight months after Travis died, Eric flew to Canada and rode his bicycle solo down the Pacific coast all the way to Mexico. He carried a backpack, pup tent, clothes, and supplies. For weeks, I tried to talk him out of this. Eric politely asked me to not say anymore unless I could be supportive.

Once again, I realized how much my boys teach me about life and letting go.

One day, after riding for two months, Eric showed up at home; tan and healthy. It was so good to have him home.

Caleb became a personal trainer. Travis was supposed to have started a new job as a personal trainer a few days after he died. With a lot of work, Caleb and a friend opened Guerilla Fitness. He enjoyed doing something he knew Travis would have done and Caleb felt peace in honoring him this way. I started going to Guerilla Fitness and Caleb became my personal trainer. He also had a tattoo done that showed he was in the same war as his brother: the "war of addiction." There are some who make it and others who do not – his brother did not.

This year, I, along with four friends, founded a grassroots organization called Disease of Addiction (DOA). Our organization helps educate the public about the Disease of Addiction. I've also been grieving the old-fashioned way: crying.

Sometimes I sit in my closet where I can be alone, and other times I drive and scream; then I feel better and go home. I'm crazy. That is all there is to it. I have also continued to paint. It is a good way to help me work through the grief, as does going on walks at Town Lake. I still attend my Al-Anon® meetings as well as a grief support group with parents who have lost children.

We wanted to do something special to remember Travis on his first Angel Date. I remembered that some of Travis's friends told me he mentioned to them that when he died, he wanted his ashes shot out of a cannon. This sounded like something that Travis would say. I thought if this was what he had wanted, then we would make it happen.

Pete worked hard and, in a few weeks, he built a life-sized cannon. On July 8, in our backyard with 65 close friends and family members, we sent Travis off with a loud blast. We shot his ashes 200 feet in the air where it exploded, scattering his ashes far and wide. I think Travis was smiling saying, "Way to Go!"

I know that once again a bit of humor helped the Morfords when we needed it the most.

So Dear Friends, know we are going to keep on going, a day at a time.

Merry Christmas; we will be back again next year.

Love,

Danni

Eric's Sojourn

—

Spring 2008

Dear Travis,

Eric trained for months to get in shape to do a bike ride down the Pacific Coast Highway. He flew to Canada to start his ride. He went north from Vancouver for a day, then headed back south. He biked 60-70 miles a day all the way down to San Diego. He met other travelers from all over the world and they rode together for a while. He went a total of about 1,500 miles. He carried his pack and bedroll and often slept by the side of the highway. Eric made it home 2 months after he left. He is so healthy and tan, and his hair is now down to his shoulders. I think this was a time for him to be alone and challenge himself and work through his loss of you.

I am grateful he is back safe and sound and stronger in all ways. I am so blessed.

All my love,

Mom

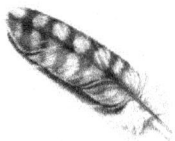

"I had a brother who was my savior.
Made my childhood bearable."
~ **Maurice Sendak**

The Cannon Shoot

—

July 2008

Dear Travis,

Your dad has been working hard on building a life-size cannon with large wooden wagon wheels. This was your wish to have your ashes shot out of a cannon. It's been a labor of your father's love, sweat and tears to honor you this way. He wasn't quite sure what to make of this request, but he knows me well enough to take me seriously.

We also worked hard in the yard to have everything looking beautiful on your first Angel Date and for the cannon shoot. We invited about 65 of your friends, your brothers' friends, and close friends of ours to join. The woman who sang Amazing Grace at your service was there to sing again.

Travis, the night was beautiful: white lights were strung in the trees, around the pool and on the stairwells. Flowers were blooming and the grass was soft and velvet green.

Your handsome dog, Tyson, was happy to have so many friends who gave him morsels of food and loved on him. I think Tyson knew this was all about you, his master and friend.

The cannon was ready to be fired and everyone began to find a place to stand. Some asked if we knew what we were doing and if we had gotten a permit? We answered "no" to both questions. That is when they stepped a bit further away from the cannon. Everyone had sparklers and was watching in anticipation. Your dad knelt down to light the fuse. We had no idea what to expect and all of the sudden, there was a very loud explosion and white billowing clouds of smoke appeared as your ashes were shot about 200 feet into the air. They burst into a fiery flame and scattered as a plane flew close by.

We were all smiling and shouting, "We love you Travis," our faces wet with tears that sparkled. The night began to overflow with so much love and memories. Your heartbeat lives on in those who know and love you.

I am sure you felt this love all the way to heaven.

Love you to heaven and back,

Mom

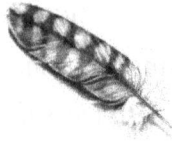

"Silently, one by one, in the infinite meadows of heaven, blossomed the lovely stars, the forget-me-nots of the angels."

~ **Henry Wadsworth Longfellow**

Guerilla Fitness

—

2008

Dear Travis,

Caleb is renting a warehouse in South Austin and turning it into a great looking gym. He painted some cool graffiti art on the interior wall, making the place pop with color. I love going to the gym and having him as my trainer. He is such a bad ass and does not cut me any slack. I need the challenge and can already feel myself becoming stronger.

We know you are here with us in spirit. Travis, please continue to watch over your brothers, the pain and loss runs deep.

Love you brown-eyed boy,

Mom

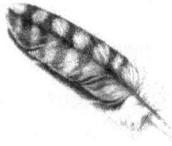

"Because brothers do not let each other wander in the dark."

~ Jolene Perry

The Christmas Letter

—

2009

Dear Friends,

What a year this has been! Eric was in a bad car wreck Labor Day weekend. He was riding with a friend, and they were hit from behind by an 18-wheeler. Eric suffered a broken neck and had to be in a brace for 4 months. The blessings in all of this are: he did not die, he was not paralyzed, and we got to spend a lot of time with him while he recovered. He is one tough kid. This put an end to his triathlons that he had been competing in for the last year.

We do have some great news. Caleb went to meet his girlfriend, Ashley, during her college studies abroad in Angers, France. Once there, he surprised her with a ring and asked her to marry him; he's such a romantic guy. We are so happy for them and are looking forward to having such a sweet, beautiful girl in the family.

Pete and I are now the owners of some land. All I can say is he and I tend to see things in a different way.

When we first saw the land, all I could see were acres of thick cactus, too many mesquite trees, and ponds that were dry from the drought. There was also an old, dilapidated trailer home. Where were the pastoral meadows? Where were the little sheep grazing in a green field of grass? Where was the Victorian house with wrap-around porch?

But when Pete saw it, his eyes glazed over, and I could almost hear the wheels turning in his head as he thought of all the fun he would have clearing the mesquite, riding the tractor, and becoming one with the land. This was not the place I had in mind; I wanted low maintenance and no years of fixing up.

I knew I was outnumbered when Eric and Caleb came to see the land. Their blue eyes glazed over just like their father's had as they began talking of hunting and bringing their friends there. I knew then, that it was a done deal. I should know by now that Pete's way of thinking and my way of thinking are going to crash headlong at times.

Thank God we have survived once again.

I have faith that Pete will turn this diamond in the rough into a thing of beauty.

So Dear Friends, we wish you a Merry Christmas; we will be back again next year.

Love,

Danni

Winter's Night

—

2009

Dear Travis,

Winter has become my favorite season. The pulse of life slows as Winter sets in. I look forward to my late-night walks with Tyson. I breathe in the frosty crystal air and the coldness stings my face. There is no cacophonous noise of locusts or birds, only the quiet, still silence of nature at rest.

Seeing the trees in Winter; their stark bare branches reaching heavenward as their roots remain strong and deep beneath the ground. Stars appear suspended on a velvet backdrop of midnight blue as they twinkle above as frozen lights. The moon ever faithful, it never disappoints, and it always reminds me of you.

The smell of wood-smoke conjures up images of our family and our time together. I savor these memories; they keep me warm. Tyson and I finish our walk; our spirits have been renewed. All is well this winter's night.

Holding you close.

Love you always,

Mom

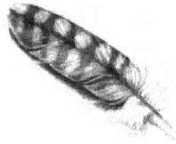

"I go to nature to be soothed and healed and to
have my senses put in order."
~ **John Burroughs**

Painting through Grief

—

2009

Dear Travis,

After you died, it took me a several months before I was able to attempt painting again. The colors I seem to work with are heavy and dark and instantly capture the feelings of grief. The brush is soaked in emotion and as it touches the canvas, my sadness finds release in the shadows. The brush strokes take on a life of their own, and the subject begins to emerge.

Painting is another way to embrace grief and sort through all that has happened. It helps me through life and guides me in the direction I should be going.

Always loving you,

Mom

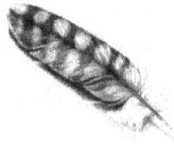

"Color is the power which directly influences the
soul."
~ **Wesley Kandinsky**

The Moon

—

2009

Dear Travis,

The past few months have been an emotional roller coaster. At times my heart actually feels like it will break. Some nights when the house is asleep, I walk by the window and gaze at the moon. I let the memories fill me with your laughter, your calls at night to say you loved me, but most of all I miss your hugs.

There is a connection I feel with you and the moon; you loved that we thought of naming you Moon Dog, and your favorite book was Goodnight Moon.

The calmness that surrounds me when I gaze up at heaven, knowing you are safe and with God and family is comforting.

I will see you again my darling son.

Always loving you,

Mom

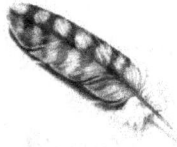

"The moon is a friend for the lonesome to talk
to."
~ Carl Sandberg

The Land Purchase

—

2009

Dear Travis,

Your dad bought a piece of property near Lockhart. It is not exactly what I had in mind, but Eric and Caleb love it as much as your dad does. The land has a lot of mesquite and cactus which is the perfect place for snakes to hide. It has an old abandoned trailer home, a barn and lots of old rusty equipment lying around.

I feel overwhelmed at the amount of work that needs to be done, but it does not seem to faze your father at all. We found the perfect area to build a fire pit; there are lots of trees and a clearing in the woods where we can sit and watch for shooting stars.

The only thing that would make it more perfect is if you were here with us.

Love you,

Mom

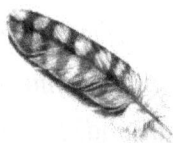

"There is a way that land speaks. Most of the time
we are simply not patient enough or quiet enough
to pay attention to the story."

~ Linda Hogan

The Christmas Letter

—

2010

Dear Friends,

Some things never seem to change – we are still as dysfunctional as ever. The last few months have been rough, to say the least. Caleb's girlfriend Ash was diagnosed with thyroid cancer.

We were a bit surprised one day when they showed up at the house and she had shaved one side of her hair off and left the other side shoulder-length. It must have been her reaction to stress. You would be proud of me. I did not react. Even though I wanted to, I did not ask what the hell she had done.

We feel hopeful that she will recover and be going strong in 2011. Please keep them in your prayers.

Tyson has a new nickname: Deer Slayer. It happened in our driveway Halloween night when Eric saw a deer and let Tyson out the front door. Eric jokingly said, "Get it." We are so grateful the neighbors did not witness "pit bull meets Bambi." We washed the blood down the driveway and hauled Bambi to the backyard before the kids showed up for trick or treat.

Eric, being resourceful, did not let the meat go to waste, the venison turned out to be very good.

Pete continues to have his mistress of 135 acres. I knew this land would steal my man. That bitch takes him away from me, always enticing him with her big spread of wide-open space. There are days when he is gone from sun-up to sun-down. There are always fences to be mended and cactus to be burned. I am glad to say I am becoming a bit countrified; I can stand right next to the cows and not climb up on the gate. We have a new calf I named Matilda. I often think of how much Travis would have liked the land.

Well, Dear Friends, it is time for me to close. We are so grateful to have you in our lives. Thank you for keeping Travis's memory alive with the memories that you continue to share with us. Your love and support help keep us going.

Travis will be forever in our hearts.

Merry Christmas from the Morfords; we will be back again next year.

Love,

Danni

Grief

—

2010

Dear Travis,

I have tried to write for hours. The room I sit in has gone from the pale yellow of morning light, to the warm gold of late afternoon. Tyson is by my side, my constant companion; he reminds me of you: handsome, beautiful brown eyes, loves to snuggle, sleep late and eat. He is strong and sensitive and loves unconditionally.

The darkness surprises me. Grief weighs me down further still. There are triggers that make grief surface to the top and boil over into night. Seeing the back of a young man's neck, the broad shoulders, dark brown hair that curls and reminds me of you.

We grieve together, Tyson for his master, and I for my son. I seek a place of solitude where I can go and sit. I breathe in the tear washed memories tattooed upon my heart and wear the veil of sadness, if only for a while.

Hearing a song, watching a movie or being in certain places brings up memories. The beating of my heart stops and then restarts. I go where my soul takes me. Grief has become my teacher.

Missing you always.

Love, Mom

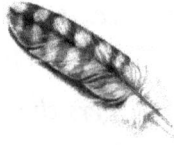

"No one ever told me that grief felt so like fear."
~ **C.S. Lewis**

The Cows

—

2010

Dear Travis,

Your dad bought some cattle for the land, and today I met the most beautiful black mama cow. She has big brown eyes and long lashes and is very friendly. There is also a huge black and white bull that weighs over a thousand pounds. We have some little cow cubes (we call them "cookies") for them to eat. They come right up next to me wanting to be fed. Their breath smells horrible and some of the cows have long, black or pink tongues that feel rough and slimy. I climbed up on the gate because I was afraid; I thought they might step on me. Tyson was with us and was very curious but kept his distance from them. I think it will take me awhile to get comfortable being a country girl.

I can picture you here with us and see your beautiful smile on your handsome face. You would love it here.

Miss you, brown-eyed boy,

Love,

Mom

"I will love you till the cows come home."
~Danni Morford

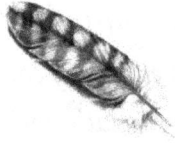

Painting the Soul Knitter

—

2010

Travis,

*Two weeks after you died, I was back in my Al-Anon®
meetings. I wanted to be with these friends; these people
who seemed the only ones who could understand the loss of
you.*

*I felt it was important not only for me to go, but also
so others could see faith in action and my belief that God
would get my family through this difficult time.*

*My painting, "The Soul Knitter," was inspired by a
woman in my Thursday group. Over time, during these
meetings, it seemed as though she knitted miles of white
yarn.*

*"The Soul Knitter" depicts an obscure figure knitting
the purest of white and intricate lace-like pattern. The yarn
begins to take shape and spills across a dark canvas of
sorrow.*

*If only I could knit you back together and wrap you in
my arms one more time, my brown-eyed boy.*

Loving you,

Mom

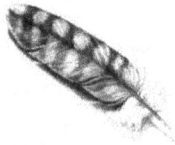

"The reason it hurts so much to separate is
because our souls are connected."
~ **Nicholas Sparks**

The Christmas Letter

—

2011

Dear Friends,

I don't know about y'all, but the holidays can be a bit stressful. That is why I am so grateful for my Al-Anon® group. We are moms and dads brought together by our need to control. Our lives had become unmanageable, because we suffer from Codependency. We are often in denial and Guilt is our middle name, and most of the time we speak before we think.

We do try and follow a strict code of ethics known as the 5 Gs:

1. *Give it to God*
2. *Get off their back*
3. *Get out of their way*
4. *Get a life*
5. *Go to a meeting*

But, the truth is, we are slow learners (and we are codependent), so most of the time we are subconsciously following our own 5 Gs:

1. *Give your addict money*
2. *Give them the car keys*
3. *Give them advice.*

4. *Give them groceries.*

5. *Get them to a meeting.*

For most of us it takes years to work The Steps. There are times when we finally say, "Let Go and Let God."

We laugh together, cry together, and comfort each other. We know how to look good under any circumstance, and the bigger the crisis the better we look. There is no greater bond than the bond between co-dependent parents.

This fall Pete, the boys, Ash, and I worked on building a fire pit in a beautiful wooded area on the land. We named it Moon Dog Forest in memory of Travis. When Travis was young, we used to joke and tell him we were going to name him Moon Dog Morford. Over the years he said that he wished we had done that.

We wanted to honor other families whose children had died. I created a mosaic on the edge of the fire pit with mementos from our children: a butterfly, ladybugs, dragonflies, a car key, an American flag, crosses, and some initials and names are just a few examples of keepsakes that lie in the mosaic. We had our first fire pit ceremony in October. About 10 couples joined, and we camped-out, built a fire, and watched for shooting stars. A new tradition has begun.

Travis's birthday was November 27th, so on a cold windy day we went to Enchanted Rock and climbed to the top. For the first time we threw some of his ashes. We had Travis's dog, Tyson, with us. It was another way we could remember his heavenly birthday.

Well, Dear Friends, it's time to say goodbye. Please know we love you and wish you a Merry Christmas; we will be back again next year.

Love,

Danni

Forget-Me-Nots

—

2011

Dear Travis,

There is a beautiful, tiny blue flower with five petals that grows in clusters. It's called a Forget-Me-Not and is symbolic of true, undying love. Forget-Me-Nots represent memories that we have of another person. A lock of your hair, your shirts, your ring, ashes and blanket are my "forget- me-nots."

My "God Moments" are the times when I have heard your voice say, "Mom," when I have found a blue jay feather, when I have seen a cloud in the shape of a cross, or when I've seen a little boy that reminds me of you. These are God's gifts to me.

Caleb told me of a dream he had about you. You had a big heart on your chest and were standing in his gym, Guerilla Fitness. You told Caleb that he looked good and that he was doing a great job.

One morning your dad showed me a cloud that looked like an arrow pointing to heaven. l loved that he shared this with me.

Eric is not quite sure what to make of all this, but I suggested he be open to the possibilities.

Maybe you can send him a sign that he can't ignore.

We will never forget you.

Love,

Mom

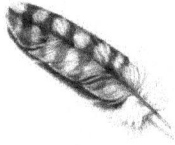

"There is a voice that doesn't use words.

Listen."

~ Rumi

The Firepit

—

October 2011

Dear Travis,

We started working on the fire pit today. We found rocks of different shapes and sizes with colors of grey, rust, and brown. Your brothers like the idea of a giant fire pit, and I want to try making a mosaic around the edge of it. Your dad stacked the rocks and cemented around them. We worked most of the day and hope to finish it in the next few weeks. I love the times we are together as a family. We are going to call this area Moon Dog Forest in memory of you.

Times like today when we are making new memories and you are not with us, weighs heavy on our hearts, but we find peace and comfort in each other.

Memories of you keep us strong.

Love you Moon Dog,

Your Family

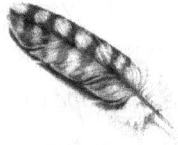

"In every walk of nature, one receives far more
than he seeks."
~ John Muir

The Fire Pit Mosaic

—

2011

Dear Travis,

This fall, I have been working on the mosaic at Moon Dog Forest. I enjoy the times when I am alone in nature. It is very soothing for me. The cows are curious, and they stop by to see what I am doing. They are such gentle creatures and help keep me company.

I have keepsakes from the other bereaved moms, and I will place them in the mosaic. I feel a closeness to their children, even though I never met them. I know their stories and how they died. I know their nicknames and can imagine their personalities. We continue sharing memories of our children. This mosaic will honor our angels and help to tell your story too.

The sounds of the forest surround me; there is beauty in the light filtering through the trees, a gentle breeze, and the rustling of leaves as a deer walks close by.

I can feel your spirit all around me when I am here. This is a very special place, this Moon Dog Forest.

You are always close by.

Love you,

Mom

"Keepsakes hold memories."
~ Danni Morford

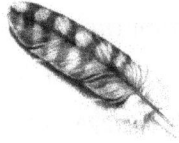

Tumbling Tumbleweed

—

2011

Dear Travis,

Our family's roots were torn apart the day you died. We have tumbled about like tumbleweed trying to find our way through grief. The days leading up to your Angel Date and your birthday always find me feeling sad, empty and restless. I want to run away where the pain cannot find me. Life keeps on going, and it has taken us in so many directions. Some that we could never have imagined.

We went to Enchanted Rock – one of your favorite places that you loved. We climbed the granite mountain breathing in the cold air and let the healing balm of nature seep into our hearts. We looked out at the view and found the perfect place to scatter your ashes. Each of us slowly released them and watched the wind carry you away. Happy heavenly birthday Travis.

Love you,

Your Family

"Sometimes I feel like a tumbling tumbleweed.
I lost my way for a while."
~ Danni Morford

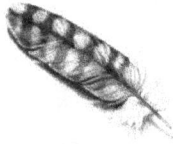

The Christmas Letter

—

2012

Dear Friends,

Each year, when I write my letter it gives me a chance to reflect on what the Morfords have been up to these past 12 months. This year, we have all been on different diets. Caleb and Ash decided to go Vegan. Eric is home from California, and he is on The Paleo diet, and Pete and I are doing a low carbohydrate diet. So, to sum it up: you have the Vegans who cannot eat anything from an animal. Paleo is based on eating fish, meat, vegetables and fruit, and our diet consists of no sugary foods or starches. I almost forgot Tyson is a vegetarian, but not by choice; we found out recently that he is allergic to meat.

I tried to be accommodating for the holiday meals and it just about did me in. Caleb and Ash go way beyond just being Vegan. They do not use a microwave; they prefer glass to plastic dishes, and they use only organic foods. And…the list goes on.

Eric wanted to eat only chickens that had been raised in Texas and he also wanted them to have been killed humanely.

I knew I had a huge Codependency relapse the day I went in search of the perfect chicken. I asked the butcher if the chickens were from Texas and if they were killed "humanely." He gave me a weird look and said, "Well lady, I know they don't sing them a lullaby." I left the store red-faced and muttering to myself, "Eric can go buy his own damn chicken."

Caleb shared some news with us; he is going to be an apprentice at Bijou tattoos on East 6th street. He will be working but not getting a paycheck for a year while he practices perfecting the art of tattoo drawing. I'm sure you can imagine how thrilled Pete and I were to hear this. On the upside, he will be able to get more tattoos for free. We did go visit the shop; it was pretty cool and not at all what we expected. Caleb has many years of sobriety and for that we are so grateful.

Eric surprised us in early spring that he would hike The Pacific Crest Trail, which starts at the border of Mexico and ends on the Washington State and Canadian border. He would be carrying a backpack weighing about 40 pounds and sleeping in a tent. He did a bit of research and got new boots and gear, but Eric being Eric (and a bit impulsive) didn't feel the need to break in his boots. Unfortunately, a couple of weeks into his hike, we received a video of him walking barefoot in the snow, feet blistered and bloody. Before cutting his trip short, he sent another picture of him leaving Travis's ashes in a beautiful spot on the trail.

Eric's feet have healed, and I'm sure they will carry him on down the road when he gets that traveling fever again.

We continue with our tradition of writing a letter to Travis on Christmas Eve and putting it in his stocking; it's another way we can keep him close and remember him at Christmas.

So Dear Friends, it's time to say goodbye.

Merry Christmas from the Morfords; we will be back again next year.

Love,

Danni

Heaven on Earth

—

2012

Dear Travis,

I dream of a place I could go; a retreat to pray, read, write, and paint. It would be built of old wood and stone and have a rustic appearance like a small chapel. There would be a few windows that would provide some natural light.

The floor would be made of concrete with an area rug to add a warm, cozy feeling. There would be a sink to wash my paint brushes, a few shelves for books, and a sturdy table to set my paints upon. I could paint when I felt inspired, not worrying about putting them away, but leave them waiting for my return.

By the window, there would be two comfortable chairs and an ottoman made of a rich tapestry of browns, rusts and golds. A quilt would drape over the chairs inviting me to linger a while longer. A few cherished objects would be placed around the room to persuade old memories to surface once again. Next to the chair, a wooden table would hold a lamp by which to read away the hours or to be alone with my thoughts – a "holiday" for my soul.

I can visualize the morning glories blooming a vibrant blue with sunlight dancing amongst the trees. Tyson, a comforting sight as he naps at my feet. All would be well in this little piece of heaven here on earth.

One day, I hope your dad will build this place for me, my home away from home. Until then, I can always dream.

Sweet dreams Travis.

Love you,

Mom

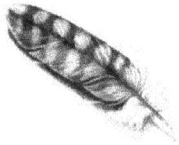

"Heaven is under our feet as well as over our heads."

~ **Henry David Thoreau**

The Cows' Names & Personalities

—

2012

Dear Travis,

I cannot believe how attached I have become to the cows! I have even named a few of them. The pretty black cow is so friendly and is always happy to see us. Her ear tag number is 3339, and this has become her nickname. It is a mouthful to say, but when I call her, she comes running. She has been curious but cautious as she gets to know me. She loves to have her head scratched and be fed cow cookies. The other is the huge bull which we named Bully. He is a gentle giant and very sweet. His head is gigantic and covered in white curly fur; his body is black, with patches of white.

There is also a red spotted cow that we call Horny because of her crooked horns. She is rather aggressive and will use her horns to move the other cows out of her way. Your dad is not allowed to sell the cows that I name, so I will have to keep naming them!

Travis, one of my favorite memories of you is the time we were at Uncle Happy's ranch for the annual dove hunt. You loved feeding the longhorns and Gus, the llama.

So many memories of you come rushing in.
Love you brown-eyed boy,
Mom

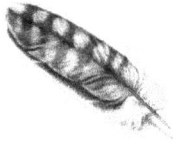

"I am not ashamed to profess my deep love for
these quiet creatures."
~ **Thomas de Quincey**

Self-Portrait of Words

—

2013

Dear Travis,

The place where the heart and emotions meet becomes the birthplace of my writing. I cannot force the words onto paper. Sometimes I have to sit and revisit the sadness and coax the pain back to life.

This contemplative time is a gift that allows my heart to surrender and be vulnerable to what my soul is trying to teach me. I continue to wrestle with grief and the guilt of not being able to keep you safe. Writing enables me to confront events in my life, finding balance, strength, and hope.

Travis, may your death not be in vain, but be a life force in helping others.

Love always,

Mom

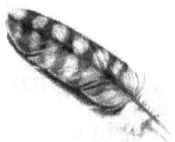

"Tears are words that need to be written."

~ Paulo Coelho

The Christmas Letter

—

2013

Dear Friends,

We started building our house out at the land. It is fun but can be stressful for someone like me, who cannot understand blueprints. It can also be stressful working with Pete, an Aggie engineer. Pete says I make no sense sometimes and that I get ahead of myself. He thinks I make more sense after I have a margarita, so I guess I will be drinking more. Pete is doing a great job. He continues to amaze me at what he can do. We are so looking forward to its completion.

Eric and Caleb are doing well. Caleb is starting to build up his clients at Bijou tattoo, and Eric is proving to be quite the entrepreneur, with some investments in real estate. I am not going to say that we are thrilled about all of Caleb's tattoos, but we are so grateful he has been sober for 9 years. I am thrilled that Eric and Pete share a love for gardening together, and also thank God that Eric no longer grows illegal crops. The father-son-duo spend a lot of time at the land growing wonderful vegetables.

Eric and Caleb have overcome their own personal struggles and are finding their own paths in ways I could never have imagined.

After Travis died, I felt the need to step out of my comfort zone and challenge myself to see what my strengths and weaknesses are. I needed to figure out what to do with the last part of my life. When I saw the movie, The Way, I received my answer of how I could push myself to the limit. The movie is about a Pilgrimage in Spain; it is known as The Camino de Santiago: a 500-mile walk across Spain, and this Camino is what I will do.

For the past 8 months, I have been training with 2 other friends who each also lost a son. We felt this would be a great way to honor our boys.

The goal is to walk The Camino in 31 days. Our date to depart is May 7th, which is my 62nd birthday.

So, Dear Friends, it is time for me to go. Know that I will be thinking of you as I walk. Please keep us in your prayers.

Love,

Danni

The Ranch House

—

2013

Dear Travis,

We decided to build the house in the back of the land overlooking the pond and the large rock formation, which looks like a giant tortoise. In the distance, a mile away, we can see only one neighboring house. There is usually a breeze in this area, which will create a perfect place to sit on the porch during the hot days.

We found some massive antique wooden beams from an old warehouse. I asked your dad to see if they were getting rid of them, and they said we could just have them! The great room is designed around the length of these beams, and we will put stamped metal on the ceiling (in between the beams) like they had 100 years ago.

The drive to the land takes less than one hour, and we hope to spend lots of time there making memories with family and friends. Building the house will take about a year, which gives me a chance to refinish some furniture that can be used there.

I miss you being here and being a part of this. I know how much you would love the peace and quiet of country life.

Love you,
Mom

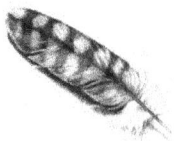

"There's no place like home."

~ L. Frank Baum

The Way

—

April 2013

Dear Travis,

In the years following your death, I have felt that God has been preparing me to be spiritually and physically fit. He has placed certain people in my life and circumstances that have gently nudged me in ways I would never have gone.

I continue to find comfort and peace in the quietness of my closet, this is where I find the answers that my soul is trying to teach me.

After I watched a movie called The Way, about a 500-mile pilgrimage across Spain, I knew I wanted to do this.

Your dad and brothers have been very supportive. I can hear you saying, "Go for it, Mom."

Love you,

Mom

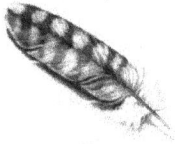

"When you walk with purpose, you collide with destiny."

~ **Ralph Buchanan**

Breaking in our Shoes

—

2013

Dear Travis,

Kate, Elda, and I have made a schedule of the days we can train, and we have also planned the details of our trip.

We are breaking in our shoes and are up to about seven miles. Our goal will be to average 17 miles per day on The Camino.

There are many different trails to walk in and around Austin. Our favorite has been at Lake Georgetown. When we finish our hike, we are usually starving. We found a place to eat called El Monumento. It has a great patio where we eat, sip margaritas, laugh, and talk about our trip.

We each have issues with our feet, but we stop and adjust our socks or apply Vaseline® to the hot spots. The time we three are together is very special. I cannot imagine doing this trip without them. Elda speaks Spanish, and she is trying to teach us a few Spanish words and phrases. It's pretty funny to hear me try to speak Spanish with my West Texas accent. I really butcher the words.

Loving you as we walk,
Mom

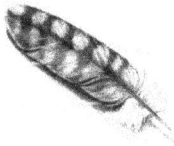

"If you want to go fast, go alone.
If you want to go far, go together."
~ African Proverb

The Christmas Letter

—

2014

Dear Friends,

I am happy to say that Pete and I celebrated our 40th Anniversary in August, and we finished building the house at the land back in October. Pete has continued to clear out acres of mesquite and cactus – the result being a wonderful view from the front porch that fills us with peace and gratitude to have this slice of heaven here on earth.

We started a new tradition of lighting sky lanterns and sending messages to Travis in heaven on clear starry nights. It is another way we keep him close to us. How much we miss that brown-eyed boy.

Sadly, this year, we found out Travis's dog Tyson, had a cancerous tumor on his leg. After taking him to the vet and discussing it with the boys, we decided to do radiation treatment. It was a rough time for all of us, especially Tyson, but he is one tough dog. This sweet pooch that we all love so much is recovering well.

I could've had a facelift for all the money we spent on Tyson's treatment, but we would not have done it any other way.

His companionship and the love and joy he continues to bring us has been worth it.

Kate, Elda, and I began our journey to complete our 500-mile walk across Spain. We first landed in Madrid and took the subway to the train station; after a 3-½ hour train-ride, we took a taxi to Roncesvalles where we would begin our walk. We were some tired but excited pilgrims.

We averaged about 17 miles a day. We endured quite a bit on our journey: we had to "thread our blisters" to help them drain, I lost 7 toenails, and we all went to the hospital at some point to receive minor medical attention. We slept in bunk beds; we carried our packs as we walked our way across Spain.

There were times we argued over who had to sleep on the top bunk and even who would carry an extra apple! Elda was the translator. She speaks excellent Spanish. Kate was the writer and did a great job of chronicling our journey and her personal experience on her blog. It's easy to find if you do an Internet search for "Kate's Kamino Blog." Every night, she was up late writing several pages and posting 30-40 photos with captions. She did all of this on the tiny screen and keyboard of her iPhone®.

During the day, I set the pace. I guess it was my long legs. We met other pilgrims from all over the world and developed our community of fellow pilgrims.

On day 31, our journey came to completion as we entered Santiago. We were greeted by bagpipes playing, greetings of fellow pilgrims as they arrived, and a ceremony blessing the pilgrims in the Cathedral of St. James. I left Travis's ashes throughout the Cathedral wherever I could find a nook, cranny, or recess. It was an emotional ending to our journey. To experience the walk with my friends and share the spirit and magic of The Camino was such a gift and one I am so grateful for.

On our last day, we took a bus to Finisterre which is known as the end of the earth. It has a beautiful view of the coastline. It was there, overlooking the ocean, that I threw some more of Travis's ashes. It was the perfect ending to a trip of a lifetime.

Thank you, Dear Friends and family, for your letters of encouragement. I read one letter each day and they lifted my spirits.

Thank you to Pete, Eric, Caleb and Ash for believing in me. May each of you find your own Way. Buen Camino.

Merry Christmas; we will be back again next year.

Love,

Danni

First Day as a Pilgrim

—

2014

Dear Travis,

After many hours of travel, we finally made it to Roncesvalles, Spain. We received our scallop shells to carry on our backpacks which identifies us as pilgrims. We stayed our first night in an old monastery and shared a room full of bunk beds with about 100 other pilgrims. I did not sleep much at all because I was so excited to see what the morning would bring. At 6:00 AM we awoke to music blaring "Good Day Sunshine!"

No amount of training could have prepared us for the steepness of the hills or the changes in elevations that we would experience.

Love,

Mom

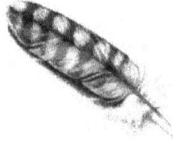

"Life begins at the end of your comfort zone."
~ **Neale Donald Walsch**

A Typical Day on The Camino

—

2014

Dear Travis,

"Walk, eat, sleep, repeat." That was the routine of our days on The Camino. It took a while for me to adjust to life as a pilgrim. Most of the hostels we stayed in had communal sleeping arrangements and bathrooms. A few, but not all, had a men's side and a women's side. There were several times we splurged and stayed at a hotel where we had a room for the 3 of us with our own bathroom, a tub, and hairdryer. This was such a luxury for us after a hard day.

Very few of the hostels had washers or dryers so we washed our clothes in an outdoor sink and hung them to dry. We spent the early evening looking for medical supplies or snacks for the next day.

People walk The Camino for many reasons: to lose weight, for adventure, loss of a loved one, loss of a job, or spiritual and religious reasons.

I love the symbolism of The Camino and the yellow arrows that help with guidance. We saw the yellow arrows painted on rocks, buildings, signs, trees, all along the roads, and throughout the towns. In certain areas you really have to pay attention, or you could easily go the wrong way, which happened to us a few times.

The Cruz de Ferro or Iron Cross stands atop a huge mound of rocks where pilgrims have left a rock with a letter, word or message written to a loved one. I left a blue jay feather, rocks with messages, and the 3-year AA chip that Shannon had given to me.

As I walked around and read the words, I became sad thinking of all the stories the messages told. I wish I had known about this pilgrimage and that we could have experienced it together as a family.

I carried each of you with me every step and every day.

Buen Camino.

Love you,

Mom

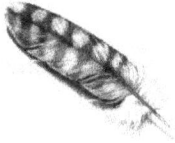

"A Pilgrim is a wanderer with a purpose."
~ **Peace Pilgrim**

Three Stages of The Camino

—

2014

Dear Travis,

There are three stages of The Camino that a pilgrim will experience. The beginning (or first) is known as "The Physical Stage." This is where you will become hyper-aware of your body and all its aches and pains. You may ask yourself why you are doing this. There were times I would zig-zag sideways when going down steep hills, in order to take the pressure off my knee and my toes. After about twelve days, my body began to adjust to the normality of blisters and to the weight of my backpack.

Next comes, the "Emotional/Mental Stage." It is also known as, "the soulless path," because of its flat terrain and lack of shade. Some of the walk is on a road next to a busy highway. The loneliness of the path is where I felt the weight of all that I carried in my heart and on my back. There were many God moments and signs along the way. The sunflowers, heart-shaped rocks, and seeing your name written on a wall reminded me of all that I was seeking.

Every day we ended our walk by saying "The Lord's Prayer." We were so grateful that we had arrived safely and were able to find a safe place to sleep that night.

"The Spiritual Stage" is the third and final stage and happens a few days before the end of the journey. During this time, I wanted to walk alone for a while and recall all the places and the magic of The Camino. I wanted to absorb every particle of my time as a pilgrim. It is hard to describe the mixed emotions I felt about re-entering the world I left behind.

Travis, I missed our family very much but the simplicity of this way of life lured me in and a part of me did not want to leave Spain. I was blessed to have a family taking care of things at home.

The Camino did provide for us, as we were able to find shelter from the wind and the rain. We found kind people who helped us when we were tired and hungry. We also found hope and peace in quaint churches and the magnificent cathedrals we entered.

Travis, it is hard to describe the exhilaration and the emotion of my time walking 500 miles across Spain. I will cherish the many memories shared with Kate and Elda.

Most of all, I will cherish being able to finish what we set out to do – honoring our boys in a unique way. I arrived in Spain looking for answers and had the time to walk and talk with God. The road was rough at times, but it led me to the answers.

I left feeling stronger, freer, and more alive than ever.

Loving you as I walked,

Mom

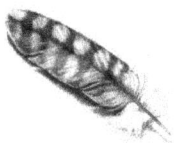

"To journey and be transformed by the journey, is
to be a Pilgrim."

~ **Mark Nepo**

Top-Ten Camino Favorites

—

2014

Dear Travis,

There were many wonderful times I experienced while walking The Camino de Santiago. This is my top ten:

1. Walking and being open to what I could learn from The Camino.

2. Being with two of the strongest, most fun and beautiful friends and experiencing the magic of The Way.

3. Our prayers at the end of each day. Being so tired and grateful for a place to rest.

4. Walking into Santiago and knowing we made it; the pain was well worth it.

5. Greeting our pilgrim family as they entered Santiago; grateful and happy they also finished safely.

6. Being greeted by bagpipes playing and seeing the Cathedral of Santiago de Compostela.

7. The ceremony and blessing of the pilgrims.

8. Carrying your ashes to the end of the earth.

9. The simplicity of life.

10. Best of all being reunited with family. Your dad brought Tyson to the airport, and I loved seeing my boys and Ash.

Our friend Butch was also at my homecoming; I remember him saying, "you are changed, I can see it in your eyes."

Last, but not least, a pedicure. OK, so that is more than ten, but they were all the best of times.

Travis, as I walked The Camino, I thought of all the traditional treatment centers you had gone to. I wish the recovery community could incorporate and adapt a pilgrimage like this into the 12 Steps. Training for the pilgrimage could be part of the recovery process. I wish I could figure out a way to make this happen.

I Love you,

Mom

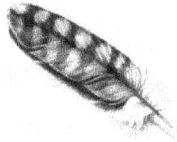

"Sometimes you find yourself in the middle of nowhere, and sometimes in the middle of nowhere, you find yourself."

~ **Unknown**

The Christmas Letter

—

2015

Dear Friends,

Next year is going to be the year of the wedding. Caleb and Ashley finally set a date for their big day! It will be June 3rd of 2016. They are so excited; it is all they can talk about.

Eric got the traveling fever again. I knew he would. He decided to move to Las Vegas to work at modeling. I jokingly asked if it was modeling with his clothes on or off. He just grinned. So that's as far as I'm going with this story. I will be glad when he finds the right girl and settles down. He was not able to be with us at Thanksgiving or Christmas; we missed him and hope he will return to Austin soon.

Pete and I have hosted several retreats at the land for The University High School, which is a high school for students in recovery. It has been a blessing getting to know these students and some of the staff. I think Travis would like that we are involved with them. I wish there had been a school like this for him.

Caleb continues his work at Bijou Tattoos, and he also continues to work as a personal trainer. Ash is a teacher's assistant in the Westlake School District and is also training to be a yoga instructor. Pete continues to build pools in Austin and raise cattle at the land. He started clearing an area next to Moon Dog Forest and is designing a labyrinth for us.

I have been working on my first mosaic, which is a tree of life. I continue to facilitate at The Christi Center for the Bereaved Parents Group.

For now, life is good at the Morford house; your friendship is such a gift to us.

Merry Christmas from the Morfords; we will be back again next year.

Love,

Danni

Writing through Grief

—

2015

Dear Travis,

For me, journaling is a journey of the heart. Since 1970, I would write my thoughts in a notebook, on scraps of paper, and sometimes in a journal. I would leave snippets of words describing my moods, thoughts, and feelings tucked away in a drawer or folder until I was ready to try and make sense of what I had written.

When I go back and read the words, they dredge up past feelings that tug on my emotions and allow the memories to resurface. This takes me to where I need to go emotionally, and my soul begins to write.

It is in feeling (and in these emotions) that I remember life with all its sadness. But more importantly, I try and remember to look for the happiness and joy that was and will be again.

I write because the words need to be written. There may be tears upon the pages, not just from sadness but also from laughter.

Life goes on.

I hope someday after I am gone, your brothers will read what I have written. If they do, they will get to know me in a way that only my writing can reveal. Maybe they too will find the gift that writing brings.

Love you darling,

Mom

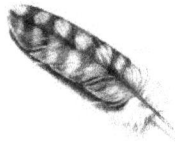

"To write is to undress the soul."

~ Danni Morford

Derailed

—

2015

Dear Travis,

The mournful wail of a train stirs a restlessness deep inside of me. I want to jump on the train and ride for a long, long time. With no care or thought of where I'm going. I just want to get away.

The train takes me to wondrous places: I see fish jumping in emerald streams; I see the highest mountains and across the deep, cobalt blue seas, to exotic foreign countries; I see forests of mammoth trees and through fields of wheat. I travel the flat West Texas Plains, hearing the coyotes howl. The sepia tone deserts of Mexico are tattooed forever on my heart.

I stop at many depots along the way: life as a daughter, sister, wife, friend, and then on to motherhood. I have times of joy and laughter, tears and sadness too. At times, the train travels through dark ebony tunnels of grief that leave me in a place of fear and anxiety. For a while, I am held hostage by my thoughts.

My heart begins to pound loudly against my chest, and there is a clanging of bells and the huffing, puffing of the train.

I am about to derail.

I feel the wind of an angel's wings lift me up, and I hear a voice saying, "follow me; trust me; everything will be alright."

I love you darling angel,

Mom

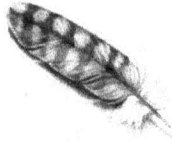

"You must learn to let go.
Release the stress."
~ **Steve Maraboli**

Memories

—

2015

Dear Travis,

I have been reminiscing about you three boys and all the fun we shared. The memories are bittersweet. Against my better judgement, I went through the many boxes of keepsakes, and tucked away, I found baby teeth, baby bracelets, locks of hair, tiny hand prints and love notes that you three gave to me. I also found the little white leather shoes you wore when you began to walk.

As I held the locks of hair, cards, and love notes, the emotions were so overwhelming, it hurt my heart and the tears began to flow.

I am grateful for the gifts of these memories that keep our love alive. These memories are like Band-aids®. They stop the bleeding for a while.

My three blessings.

Love,

Mom

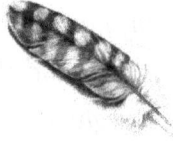

"Memory is the diary that we all carry with us."
~ **Oscar Wilde**

The Christmas Letter

—

2016

Dear Friends,

Caleb and Ashley had a beautiful and fun wedding with family and close friends. They surprised the guests with a presentation of their wedding dance for which they had practiced for months. Eric gave a heartfelt toast to the bride and groom that had us all laughing and crying.

There was a delicious wedding cake, Vegan burritos, and there was even Vegan wine and beer! I'm glad Ashley had the wedding she'd always dreamt of. It was a night to cherish as a family, knowing that Travis, our brown-eyed boy, was there with us in spirit. He would be so proud of his brothers.

The happy couple went to Thailand for their honeymoon. Two weeks into it, Caleb became very sick with a high fever. He was hospitalized and treated for Dengue Fever, which he contracted from a mosquito bite. Pete and Ashley were on the phone with the airline for days. Finally, Pete was able to get their revised departure date worked out. Caleb had to stay an extra four days to regain his strength in order to safely make the flight home.

I am so thankful for Ashley and how she took such good care of Caleb when they were so far away from home.

The two of them have been through a lot over the years. With Ashley having thyroid cancer, Caleb enduring the loss of Travis and then getting Dengue Fever on the honeymoon! Hopefully, the vow of "in sickness and in health" has run its course.

Caleb and Ashley are settling in to married life. Ashley is still teaching at the elementary school and is a yoga instructor on the weekends. Caleb is building up his clientele at Bijou tattoos. He no longer has the gym but continues to be my trainer twice a week at our home, along with 3 of my friends.

Eric is back in Austin living in the heart of downtown. He is working on some start-up companies. One of these has Vegan, organic, beauty products, which is named FoxyBoxy. He is disciplined with his workouts and eats healthily. He has no fear of going where his heart leads him.

Pete continues building pools but hopes to take on fewer jobs in the next few years. He enjoys time at the land where there is always something to be done. He is starting to relax and can sit on the porch and read a book. He has become a great cook and enjoys cooking for friends and family. I am once again training with Kate and Elda. We plan to do another pilgrimage in 2017.

Travis's dog, Tyson is now 13 years old. He has trouble hearing, has arthritis, and sometimes needs help going up and down the stairs. He still enjoys going on walks, taking naps, and being the family dog. I help him get up on the bed at night where he likes to snuggle. Over the years, Pete has gotten used to Tyson sharing our bed. I love Pete for that.

Eric, Caleb and Ashley have been our anchor throughout the years since Travis died. They have supported us with acts of kindness and patience and loved us when we needed it the most. More importantly, for today, they are enjoying life. For this I am so grateful.

Merry Christmas everyone; we will be back again next year.

Love,

Danni

Tree of Life Mosaic

—

2016

Dear Travis,

I finished the mosaic that will hang on the front porch out at the land. I had my work area set up on the porch downstairs where it was protected from the rain and sun. Tyson loves being outside with me as I work. There were days when I would work for eight or more hours. I would get lost in the process of creating.

This mosaic is a Tree of Life, which I hope tells our family's story. It is three feet by five feet, and your dad framed it in steel. The main focus is a tree with bare branches and deep roots. The background is a night sky with a giant yellow moon and some stars.

As I worked on this mosaic, some of the objects I incorporated are: your AA chip, shells from our family beach trips, marbles that you and your brothers played with, a few crosses, and the serenity prayer. I used slate, rocks, small pebbles, glass, and pieces of a broken mirror. All of these pieces added texture of rough and smooth layered edges.

Travis, I also mixed some of your ashes in with the grout and shed tears as I worked to honor and remember family we have loved and lost.

This Tree of Life is filled with memories and our sorrow is also buried deep within. Family is what keeps us strong and shelters us through life's storms. I love to look into the broken pieces of mirror and see my father's nose, my mother's eyes, and know that our ancestors live on in our family.

Loving you,

Your Family

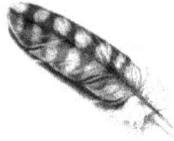

"We are mosaics – pieces of light, love, history & stars – glued together with magic, music & words."

~ **Anita Krishan**

Gratitude

—

2016

Dear Travis,

When I am having a hard day, I know it's alright to let the sadness in. But, more importantly, I know that I cannot stay in the sadness too long. Grief is hard work. It wreaks havoc with your sleep, your memory, and it can make you physically sick. Even when I do not feel like working out or meeting with a friend for coffee, I go anyway and usually leave feeling better.

It is important to remind myself of all that I have to be grateful for. I am grateful for your dad, who has been my safe place throughout the years. He has loved me when I'm not very lovable, he cares for me when I'm sick, and being with him helps growing old be a bit easier.

Eric, Caleb and Ash, give us the gift of their presence, kind actions and loving words. So many thoughtful acts of kindness over the years. It is comforting to see glimpses of you in them.

I think what I'm trying to say is, I am very blessed to have each one of you in my life.

Love you darling,

Mom

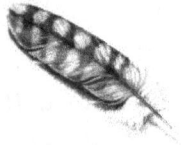

"Gratitude elevates our moods and fills us with joy."

~ Sara Avant Stover

Forever Changed

—

2016

Dear Travis,

Your death had a great impact on our marriage. All the existing issues that we were dealing with before your death, were exacerbated when you died. This August your dad and I will have been married for forty-two years.

During our years of marriage, we have enjoyed many beautiful sunsets and sunrises. We have also weathered many storms along the way. Droughts of no communication, time of anger, and hurt feelings on both parts. The worst to ever test our marriage was the day you died.

The percentage for divorce after the death of a child is extremely high. Our saving grace was The Christi Center. That is where we found a safe place to learn about and share our grief.

Not one of us will ever be who we were before you died, but we are definitely better together.

Love you,

Mom

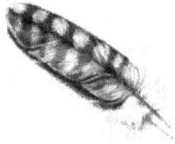

"Love never dies."

~ Unknown

The Christmas Letter

—

2017

Dear Friends,

Eric discontinued FoxyBoxy and has capitalized on his web skills to create an online wholesale natural medicine business.

Caleb and Ash celebrated their one-year anniversary and were able to purchase their first home. We spent many weekends working in the yard and painting some of the bedrooms of their new home. We enjoyed having Thanksgiving dinner at their home this year.

Pete and I worked on an area near Moon Dog Forest to build a labyrinth. In May, we plan to have the students from University High School finish laying the rocks as part of their yearly retreat.

Kate, Elda and I were unable to do another hike together as we had planned, but we still enjoy the times we get together and hike in Austin.

Easter weekend, Eric surprised us with a parasail he had purchased for the family to try out. The facts that we have no large body of water to sail over, that none of us like heights, nor have any experience doing this, made no difference to him.

Eric, being very persuasive, got everyone involved in helping him with the parachute. It was terrifying to see him way up in the sky being pulled by the ATV. The cows were running after him while a plane kept circling the land to see what was happening. Eric made it look so easy, so Caleb, Ash and I parasailed too. Wow! It was so scary, but so much fun.

Pete did not fare so well. There was a problem with the rope and he never made it off the ground. The wind shifted, and he was dragged sideways and hurt his shoulder pretty badly. We didn't have a sling, so I used a sheet for his arm and put ice on his shoulder. This is probably one of the craziest things our family has done, and we are very grateful to have survived another year.

It has been ten years since Travis died, so we decided to have another cannon shoot at our land. On July 8th we invited a few close friends of the family to come to the land and celebrate his life. We spent the day and on into the evening being together and sharing stories and memories of Travis. It was a beautiful evening to shoot his ashes out of the cannon and honor him again that night.

We wish you a Merry Christmas; we'll be back again next year.

Love,

Danni

Country Life

—

2017

Dear Travis,

Your father and l are extremely grateful for the land and the opportunity to build a home to share with our family and friends. It has been a healing place where our family can enjoy the simple pleasures of cooking meals, playing games, and picking vegetables from the garden.

The rocking chairs on the porch invite us to sit and enjoy the view of the pond and the cows grazing in the field that your father worked so hard to clear. Sharing the land is what it's all about.

Travis, with all my blessings, my heart still hurts and wishes you were here with us.

Love you forever,

Mom

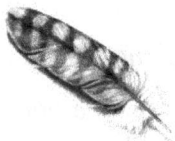

"Those we love and lose are always connected by heartstrings into infinity."
~ **Terri Guillemets**

Strength of Family

—

2017

Dear Travis,

When I heard that Eric had been in a bad car wreck, I felt such panic and fear knowing that I could not go through losing another child. I felt the same panic when I got the call from Ashley, when Caleb was hospitalized in Thailand with Dengue Fever. Each one of us has felt sadness, depression, stress, panic, and anxiety over the years since you died.

What I want you to know Travis, is that grief in all its ugliness has not made our family weak.

Our strength comes from what we carry inside of us: your spirit, our faith, and our family's love.

We will always love you,

Mom

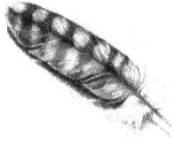

"Pain is real, but so is hope."
~ Unknown

The Christmas Letter

—

2018

Dear Friends,

In October, Caleb and Ash surprised us with the news that they are having a baby! We are so happy for them and look forward to this next part of our life.

Both the boys have their own businesses. Eric rents a warehouse in South Austin and employs several workers to help with his online business. Caleb and a partner opened their own Tattoo shop which is also in South Austin. It is called, Red Stag Tattoo.

Ash continues as a nanny for several kids and also helps to tutor them. She is learning about wood fired ceramics and has made some beautiful pieces.

Pete retired from building pools, which has allowed him time to help the boys with their projects. He also has more time to get a lot done out at the land.

I have had the pleasure of working on a mosaic with the students at the sober high school (University High School). They are so creative, and I enjoy spending time with them.

Our family enjoys being together at the land. The kids introduced us to several new card games; Cards Against Humanity and You've got Crabs. I had never heard of some of the words and kind of wish that was still the case. We did have fun and laughed a lot.

Our sweet dog, Tyson died on Good Friday, he was fifteen years old. We miss him dearly. What a comfort and joy he was to us. I picture him with Travis in heaven. Oh, what a reunion they must've had!

I have been writing our Christmas Letter for 14 years and can honestly say that the Morfords are still far from normal. You know what? It's okay. I love that we were daring enough to parasail over the land, not knowing what in the heck we were doing and that we survived. I love that we go hunting for rattlesnakes before they can find us.

Most of all, I love that Travis lives on in each of us. We hold on to memories of our time with him while creating new traditions and memories. Life is ever changing.

Thank you all for sharing it with us.

Merry Christmas from the Morfords; we'll be back again next year,

Love,

Danni

You're an Uncle!

—

2018

Dear Travis,

Caleb and Ash invited us over for dinner and surprised us with a gift. When we opened the bag, we unwrapped a darling coffee mug with a drawing of a hand holding a pregnancy test, a cute little baby, and the words that said, "We're having a BABY! Coming summer 2019."

It took a few moments for it to register with your dad and me, but when it finally registered, we were so excited! Caleb and Ash were beaming and, of course, we all had tears in our eyes, and they secretly captured the moment on a GoPro® camera. Eric had other plans that evening and was not there for the surprise.

Travis, this baby will know who you are and over the years will read your letters, see pictures of you, and hear stories from all of us. Life can be so bittersweet at times.

Love you,

Mom

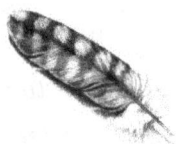

"Every family has a story. Welcome to ours."
~ **Unknown**

Missing Tyson

—

2018

Dear Travis,

For several months, we could see that Tyson was becoming frail, and we knew he would not be with us much longer. He still followed me from room to room, but it was hard for him to stand up and walk. Each time your brothers and Ash would leave Tyson, they would always say their goodbyes knowing they might not be at the house when he died.

One morning we knew it was time to have the vet come to the house. Tyson was tired and ready to be with you. I could see it in his big brown eyes. Your dad and I held him and told him how much we loved him. I thanked him for being such a sweet loving companion and part of our family. I whispered and kissed him and said he would be with you soon. My heart was breaking, it felt like I lost you again.

The house has felt so empty without Tyson greeting us at the door and being there to go on our walks together. Most of all, I miss him being with me in my closet as I write.

The neighbors gave us a memorial stone when Tyson died. We placed the special stone near the fountain by the porch out at the land. I have also placed heart-shaped rocks and other little things there to remind me of the two of you. I am glad I have the painting of him, which hangs with my other paintings.

I remember when you died, Tyson grieved for you for many months. It comforts me to know you two are together again, and he is giving you doggy kisses.

Love you, my brown-eyed boy,

Mom

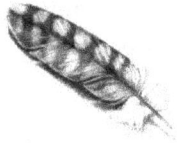

"A dog is the only thing on earth that loves you
more than he does himself."

~ **Josh Billings**

Letters to Baby

—

2018

Dear Travis,

My first journal began in the Fall of 1970 when your dad and I began dating. I would usually write at night after our date. I continued for the four years he and I dated. After we were married and I found out I was pregnant with you, I started keeping a journal and wrote regularly for the entire nine months.

When Eric was born several years later, I kept a journal for the first year of his life. By the time Caleb came along, I did not have time to write. I have always felt a bit guilty that he will not have a journal. I began writing to the new baby. I figure this will be my way of making amends to Caleb.

Dear Baby,

Oh my gosh, you are the topic of all our conversation. Your mom and I spend hours talking about the nursery and your birth. What fun it will be to have a baby in the family!

Your mom is the picture of health and grows more radiant every day, and your dad compares your size to a seed or fruit. Your parents have read a ton of books and watched lots of videos about what you look like at each stage; your dad got a bit weirded-out when they said you had a tail and gills, but it is nice to see them be so involved with every stage of your development.

They have decided not to find out whether you are a boy or a girl, so you will be a big surprise! My friends are so excited for us to experience being grandparents. I can't wait to meet you, and I'm excited to see how our family evolves.

Love you

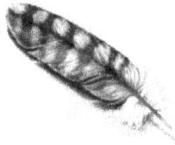

"Our family is a circle of strength and love.
With every birth and union, the circle will grow."
~ Unknown

Afterword

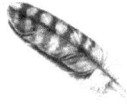

Dear Friend,

I hope this book helped you and that it helps connect others who have experienced chaos, fear and sadness that comes along with the disease of addiction. I want you to know you're not alone. Most of all try, when you can, to laugh through the tears, because humor is what has really gotten me through some of the toughest times. I would like this message to stay with you long after you have finished this book.

I also want you to realize everyone handles pain, struggle and grief differently, and my hope for you is that in The Letters you will find your own answers and they can help guide you.

One thing that helps me is to give back and bring about awareness to this horrible disease. I hope my story will help eliminate the stigma and shame that makes it so hard for an addict to recover.

Love,

Danni

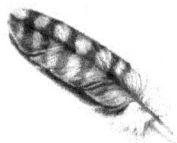

"Awareness is powerful.
Tell your story.
Here's the rest of mine…"

Epilogue
One Step Forward, Two Steps Back

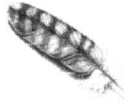

Being a wife and mom of three boys kept me very busy. I loved being a stay at home mom and am grateful I was able to do this. Life was going well at our house until 1993 when our oldest son, age twelve, started experimenting with marijuana and, eventually, went to alcohol and stronger drugs. Our family was entering into a struggle with a disease we knew very little about. We became so focused on our oldest son. So much so, that we did not see what was happening with our other two boys.

By the year 2000, it was total chaos at our house. In September of that year, our oldest went to treatment in Minnesota; this was hard for our family. We missed him so much but felt he would be in a safe place and would be able to receive help for his addiction. This would be the first of many treatment centers and family weeks at rehab we would go to over the years.

The Disease of Addiction was beginning to affect our whole family and creating a lot of stress in our marriage. I had resisted going to Al-Anon® meetings for years because I thought I'm not the one with the problem. As time went by, I became more obsessed with trying to fix the boys: I snooped in their rooms, I constantly gave unsolicited advice, and I finally became so miserable, I decided that I should try Al-Anon®. At my first meeting, some members shared they had been attending meetings for 20 years or more. I thought, no way was I ever going to be here 20 years from now. Never, say never.

Step 1. We admitted we were powerless over alcohol, that our lives had become unmanageable.

This is a very important step and one that I find myself going back to over the years. Unfortunately, I have relapses just like the addicts in my life. At times, I did not sit quietly, I did not think before I reacted, and I slipped back into old behavior of being fearful, controlling, and obsessive (about the boys' activities). I lost my peace and let anxiety slip in. I realized, "working the steps," as we say, is just as vital for me and my relationships with my family, as it is for my addicts. This is a family disease, and it would be years later before I could see what role I played in all the chaos.

We were all together often as a family, going on vacations to the beach every year and spending time with aunts, uncles, and cousins for holidays and all the festivities of the seasons. Pete and I were involved with the boys' sports and at their schools. But, the disease of addiction was always lurking about.

It was not easy to find a therapist who truly understood addiction, and if medicines were prescribed, sometimes things were made worse. I was beginning to lose confidence in doctors and therapist and also in myself. I was also upset my husband would not go to meetings with me. I became angry and resentful. We did not agree about certain things concerning the boys. Hurtful words were said and unfortunately, the boys witnessed this at times.

Step 2. *Came to believe that a power greater than ourselves could restore us to sanity.*

This step makes me so aware of how much I crave a peaceful life for myself and my family. All the steps continue to be a part of my life. I hear helpful slogans such as, "Let Go and Let God," "Easy does it," and "Keep it Simple, Stupid." I often repeat The Serenity Prayer, which always helps to quiet my mind.

Al-Anon® has played a big part in my education about this disease. It's the one place where I feel safe sharing my story. Over the years, this group has become a second family to me. I continue to benefit when I hear others share their stories and when I witness the hope and strength found in the meeting rooms.

Step 3. *Made a decision to turn our will and our lives over to the care of God as we understood Him.*

I was a slow learner with this step. As much as I want God's will in my life, sometimes I catch myself telling Him how and when I want it done. I'm glad God has a sense of humor and understands my weaknesses.

Our youngest was the first to ask to go to treatment; he was ready to change the downward path he was on with the abuse of drugs and alcohol. He went to treatment, and this would be the first time he would not be with us for Thanksgiving or Christmas. He was only 17 and would be living in another state for 6 months. Pete, the older two boys, and I made the trip several times to go and see their brother. This disease is a destroyer of lives and we certainly felt its effects, but in a strange way we became closer because of some of the hardships we experienced together.

Step 4. *Made a searching and fearless moral inventory of ourselves.*

At every meeting, we read The Twelve Steps, and I would hear members mention their experience of working Step 4. Being honest with myself about my strengths, weaknesses and defects of character was going to be some hard, soul searching work. This was not something I looked forward to doing, so I put if off for a few years. When I was finally ready to get to work, I began to honestly look at my actions over the years and was not too happy with what I saw.

Working this step allowed me to see how my behavior played such a significant part in the chaos of my family. I have become more aware of my thoughts and actions and try to catch myself before I relapse into old behavior. Usually, it's just a matter of me keeping my mouth shut and asking God for help.

Step 5. *Admitted to God, to ourselves, and another human being the exact nature of our wrongs.*

This is a humbling step to do. It required me admitting my deepest secrets and shame to God, to myself, and to another person. For me, telling God was easier because I knew Him as a loving God, but to admit these things to myself was not so easy. I had to honestly admit how I tried to justify my actions and manipulate situations. The times I spoke hurtful words, reacted out of anger or fear, and seeing the damage it has done was not pleasant at all. To share this with another person, trusting them to never share what was said, and hoping they would not judge me was a huge step for me.

I asked a good friend, with whom I was comfortable, if I could share my Step 4 with her. Sharing with her was still hard to do but it was a relief to get rid of the baggage I had been carrying for years.

Over a period of several more years, I worked Step 4 again and again. The last time I did it, I shared with about 8 of my Al-Anon® friends. We met once a week for about a year and a half and called ourselves "Step Sisters." I realized I still had more to get honest about and how grateful I was to have had another opportunity to work on myself.

Step 6. *We were entirely ready to have God remove all these defects of character.*

I had to accept myself just the way I was and also have the willingness to let go of all that was keeping me from a healthy life. I had to trust God to do for me that which I could not do for myself. I was not capable of ridding myself of these defects of character. I had become a bit too comfortable with some of my defects and not sure I really wanted to let go of them. Silly me, nothing good ever came from being angry or obsessing over something I couldn't control. Didn't I know that yet?

When I first started going to Al-Anon®, my family wasn't too sure how this was going to affect their lives. Over time, the meetings and groups helped me understand what my family was going through in the AA meeting rooms and we were able to discuss the steps. There were times when they suggested I should go to a meeting and my husband would give me a dollar. Having a sense of humor helped.

Step 7. *Humbly asked Him to remove our shortcomings.*

This step is where I had to take action and learn to be still and ask God for help. I then had to trust Him enough in all areas of my life. Over the years, the disease of addiction brought me to my knees more times than I can count. I knew that with this disease, my boys would either recover, go to jail, or die.

Surrendering to God was not giving up but it was putting my faith in Him knowing that he would help get my family through whatever happened.

Step 8. Made a list of all persons we had harmed and became willing to make amends to them all.

Wow. Another difficult Step for me to do. Working this Step served as a gentle reminder for me to refrain from doing or saying something I would later regret and have to apologize for. The suggestion in Step 8 is to ask ourselves the following questions before saying or doing something: "Is it kind? Is it necessary? Is it helpful?" Usually, I cannot go wrong if I practice this.

Step 9. Made direct amends to such people wherever possible, except when to do so would injure them or others.

Early on in joining and working The Steps, I did not embrace Step 8 or 9. I was still too angry, and it was not very healthy to think about the pain my words and actions caused others or to even think about how my own words and actions had affected me.

In recent years, I worked more on changing my behavior, and over time I was slowly learning to make amends to those I have harmed.

Step 10. *Continued to take personal inventory and when we were wrong promptly admitted it.*

At times, I have relapsed because I got too comfortable and became lazy about going to my meetings. I began to realize that the times when I was not working the program, were the times when my anxieties and old behaviors would creep back in. The slogan, "It works if you work it" is so very true.

A practice I have found to be helpful is this: at the end of the day, I think about ways I acted or things I said. Then, I think about how I could have possibly done something differently (better, with more thoughtfulness and kindness). Holding myself accountable is important.

Step 11. *Sought through prayer and meditation to improve our conscious contact with God as we understood Him, praying for knowledge of His will and the power to carry that out.*

When I have practiced Step 11 throughout the day, I realize my life is much more peaceful. It is important for me to stay physically, mentally, and spiritually healthy. I do this by going on walks, exercising, and making sure I do not over-commit myself.

Step 12. *Having had a spiritual awakening as a result of these steps, we tried to carry this message to others, and to practice these principles in all our affairs.*

A friend of mine was the essence of carrying this Step 12 message on to others. She is the one who slowly and gently nudged me to going to my first meeting. She helped me with The Steps and was always open and honest in sharing her story. We have laughed and cried a lot together over the years.

I want to continue doing for others what she so kindly did for me. I have been in Al-Anon® 18 years and have been a sponsor to other women over the years. This has been a gift to me, because I learn from them and it serves as a reminder of where I was before. So much for "I'll never be here 20 years from now!"

The Aftermath

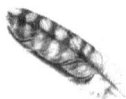

The disease of addiction was relentless in trying to take down our family. Our life was consumed with round-the-clock calls: jail, car accidents, emergency room visits, and therapist appointments. The stress and heartache we experienced as a family, at times, left us barely standing. Addiction is a disease that causes things to break: the law, trust, friendships, and marriages.

We had a small window of opportunity when all the boys were doing well. We went to Disney World in 2005 and then in 2006 our family spent 3 weeks traveling in Europe. These were the first times in a long while that we had our family together sharing time that didn't involve visiting for Family Week at a treatment center. We almost bought into the illusion that we were a normal and functioning family.

On July 8, 2007 I received the phone call no parent ever wants to receive. Our oldest son was dead. He died at age 25 from an accidental overdose. The disease that our son had fought for so many years had now proved to be much too strong for him.

The grief we felt over the death of our son and seeing our other two boys going through such grief was almost *unbearable. I wondered how we were going to survive this awful nightmare.*

But, as you can see, we did survive, and we survived because of our faith in God and with the help and prayers of so many that were there with us in the weeks and months that followed. Something I had heard years ago about how Al-Anon® and its members would get me through any loss or situation was true. They did just that and have continued to be a source of strength for me and for my family.

After our son died, my boys and their friends told me how tired they were of losing friends to addiction. I made a promise to them and to Travis, that I would do whatever I could to raise awareness about this disease.

Six weeks after Travis died, I founded a grassroots organization along with 4 of my friends. We named it Disease of Addiction (DOA). We held the first meeting at the high school my boys graduated from and about 400 people attended. We had a distinguished panel of experts in the field of addiction who spoke and answered questions from the audience. Some of our son's friends helped with this event. We continued this for several years at other schools and met with the Austin Independent School District Board Members to discuss the prevalent use of drugs and alcohol among students.

Four months after Travis died, I attended my first grief support meeting at a place in Austin called The Love of Christi for parents who have lost a child. They also have meetings for the loss of spouse, sibling- and friend-loss, and relatives of those who have been left behind by suicide.

Three months after my first meeting, my husband started attending the Dads' group. We both feel our marriage may not have survived if we had not sought help. These years later, we are still keeping our promise to Travis, his brothers and their friends: in addition to founding DOA, we have served on the Board at The Christi Center and have also been group facilitators (for both the moms' and the couple's groups). I have served on the Advisory Board of Austin Recovery. Also, both Pete and I are involved with University High School (UHS), the first safe sober high school in Austin, Texas.

We believe if UHS had been available to our family, Travis would be alive today. Beyond high school organizations, we are also connected to the first sober fraternity in the Austin area (Alpha/180).

In being active with groups and organizations like this, we can help others with addiction and share our story in an effort to help others. It is also another way we can honor our son's memory. We chose to be open about our family's struggle and hope that lives will be saved because of our honesty. We would also like to save another family from experiencing the loss of someone they love to this disease.

No one chooses to be an addict – you can hate the disease while still loving the addict. Try to talk as a family when discussing an issue related to the addiction and try to always do it with grace and love.

Be kind: No shame. No blame.

An addict fights for their life every day in ways we can never understand. While it is hard to watch your addict struggle, imagine how hard it is to live with addiction. If your friend or family member needs treatment, try to research several centers and visit beforehand, so you have options before the crisis happens. Keep communications open. Ask each other how to find solutions, as a family. It's a family disease, so don't forget to look at yourself, monitor and modify your behavior, and work on you in this process.

After losing Travis, what helped me the most was my passion to help others, share our family's story, and to keep our son's memory alive. Also, over the years, I have received letters from friends and strangers saying how their child is alive today because we shared our story. This helps our hearts and lessens the sadness, because if one life is saved, our son did not die in vain.

Travis' Letters

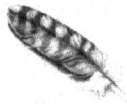

Travis, your words are powerful, and they live on.

Dear Shannon,

I'm sorry to hear about your current circumstances, but if you think about it, things could always be worse. I hope you can use this time for self-reflection and turn this into a positive thing. Sorry, I know you're thinking, "Fuck you, Travis (A.K.A. Captain Hypocrite)", but I believe you have a lot of potential in whatever you may choose. You are faced with two paths and you've experienced both, but it seems like enough is enough and its time for us as in me and you just to grow up and become so called productive members of society. I have done a lot of thinking about what I want in life and the direction I was headed; was the life I'm trying to leave behind. I've been sober 2 weeks and things are good for me.

Well man I just wanted you to know I am praying for you all the time.

Hang in there Shannon
Love, your friend,
Travis Morford

Hey Bud,

I got really strung out and just as I had anticipated the pain got really bad. It was bad enough to reach out for help. I was eating tons of Xanax, smoking crack, shooting heroin, coke and speed. Boy, shit piled up fast and I am still feeling some of the effects, scar tissue detox. Something good came from it all, and that was I went back to AA, and I started working the steps again. My family isn't speaking to me right now which hurts, but thats my fault and I'll have to suffer the consequences. I have faith that if I stay sober everything else will work itself out.

I'm sorry I haven't written in a while, my priorities got a bit screwed up, but hopefully I am back on track now. I just want you to know your still in my prayers and if you don't mind please keep me in yours, God knows I need them. Well man hang in there and remember, "thou will, not mine, be done", it's harder than it sounds but sometimes thats just the way it is.

keep your head up and remember you still have people who care.

Love,

Travis

Hey Man,

What's up? I'm sorry to hear about your Grandfather, but he's no longer in pain and he lived a pretty good life. Between me and you, my prediction of pot leading me to harder things came true. It started out when I spent a grand on some bars to help me quit smoking pot, which I did, but instead I've been eating bars, morphine, and shooting coke and smack for the past 3 days. And I'm not gonna lie to you, I had an awesome time for the first

30 minutes to an hour or so, but after the initial buzz subsided, the old feeling of the insanity of addiction quickly returned, and I feel like the pain I was telling you about in my last letter has begun to show its evil face when I look in the mirror.

I have too much time on my hands right now and I believe that has a lot to do with it. So, before I sink any lower, I think I'll try going back to A.A. I'll let you know how it turns out. I haven't used today and that's a start.

Write me back and let me know how you're doing with everything.

Hang in there, I'm praying for you always.

Your friend,

Travis Morford

Dear Luci,

I'm sorry to hear of your husband, Shannon's recent passing. I know that after living in matrimony for as long as the two of you had been, it will be difficult for you to not hear his sophisticated, but raspy voice around the house. But for a strong woman like you, it won't take long to fill the void in your heart and soul that your husband once and in a way always will fill. Just cherish the time that Shannon and you spent loving each other and realize that he's

waiting for you in an afterlife
of infinite proportions compared
to our time we spend here on
earth. So, every time you get
sad, angry, hurt, depressed, or
just lonely, all you need to
do is remind yourself that
Shannon's looking down from
heaven on you and I'm almost
positive he would want you to
mourn him to a certain extent,
that is healthy, not harmful
to you. Instead, maybe you
could celebrate the life that
the two of you spent together
just through cherishing keepsakes
that he gave you while he was
alive.

And know that one day (many years from now), the two of you will be joined once again in an infinite state of holy matrimony in a place so glorious that you'll wonder why ya'll couldn't have just both died sooner (just jokin'). But I just wanted to let you know that you and your family are in my prayers always and if there's anything that I can help you with, please don't hesitate to call me — (512)944-XXXX)

All my Love and Prayers,
Travis Morford

Dear Roberta,

I wanted to thank you for the help you gave me a few weeks back. Although it was somewhat embarrassing, I was truly grateful for your help. I want you to know it was not in vain, I went back to AA and got a sponsor, who is taking me through the steps, and because of this and the grace of God, I have close to three weeks sober.

I realize that I face a long road ahead but faith keeps me confident that I can succeed if I keep doing the right thing.

Anyway I hope you can understand how much you helped me and that you will always have a special place in my heart. I truly believe that it's people like you, who make life on earth that much more beautiful. If I can ever help you or your loved ones please don't hesitate to ask.

Love,

Travis

Dear Shannon,

Once again I have to apologize for not writing sooner. I think it was easier to write you when I was still getting high. I think the drugs kept me from realizing that I'm equally as deserving of incarceration as you and it's scares me. In the past eighteen days (how long I've been clean), I've had a lot of realizations, but the one that rings the loudest is that if I keep using, I'm destined to live a miserable life and die angry and bitter and alone.

The thought of that is unbearable to me. So, because of these things I've been going to the 5:30 Westlake meeting almost every day, and for the first time in months I feel joy and inner peace, something I hope you are experiencing as well, at least as much as you can, given your circumstances.

I was driving down S. Lamar the other morning and I saw two older men in their 70's or 80's maybe just enjoying a morning stroll and they looked overwhelmed with happiness like they were so grateful to be alive that they were going to take advantage of every moment that they had left. This made me think of you and me someday shooting the shit old and wise from experience.

Well enough of that, I just thought it was cool. Any way I ran into a friend at a meeting last Sunday. He sends his regards and hopes your doing well. He has 8 months clean. It was really cool to see him doing well after what happened to his brother, who o.d. from heroin and died. I don't know what I would do in that position, I would hope I could stay sober.

I guess thats all thats going on in my life now, its

kind boring but it beats the chaos I left behind. Hang in there Shannon I know this is far from easy on you, but I truly believe God has a greater plan for us and we can't fulfill it if were strung out, dead or incarcerated. So, don't get down on yourself and realize this too, shall pass.

Much Love,

Your friend, Travis

Let me know if I can help in any way— seriously.

Guarantee

What can you count on?
What can you be sure of?
Who can you trust?
What will happen?
Nothing is for sure.
Will tomorrow come?
Or shall we be done?
Done with life
Done with death
Done with oneself
Done, done with it all
Or not, maybe it will be
alright

But if we can't count on
Life
What can we count on?
I'll tell you what
There being only 1
No matter how hard you try
No matter how fast you run
No matter how good you are
Or how long you have trained
You cannot escape it
The only thing in your life
The only guarantee
That guarantee is Death
The inescapable fate of life
The one thing you may count
on,
The one undodgeable fatal
obstacle

Some may have fear for such
an event
But I,
I look at it as another
beginning of life
A life that I look forward
to
Life with no destruction
Immortal life
Life with no beginning or end
Life that lives on forever
Life with a complete state of
peace
No Hate
Just Love
Love toward oneself
Love towards all
Not remembering yet not
forgetting

Life so beautiful and so
abstract
So much so that any mortal
being could not handle such
greatness
This is your one guarantee
Look at it as an inspiration
Don't fear it.
Death is the only guarantee.

"I know you're thinking 'fuck you, Travis aka Capt. Hypocrite, but I believe you have a lot of potential."

"I hope you can use this time for self-reflection and turn this into a positive thing."

"To be honest, my biggest problem right now is smoking pot."

"I want to be sober, but I am currently not experiencing enough pain to put more effort into my own sobriety."

"I guess I'll either get it sooner or later or die trying. Can you tell I need a meeting?"

"It's sad that it takes such an extreme situation to make us realize how necessary it is to change our ways."

"Enough is enough. It's time for us to grow up and become so called productive members of society."

" ... been sober for two weeks and things are good."

"So, before I sink any lower, I think I'll try going back to AA. I haven't used today, and that's a start."

About the Author

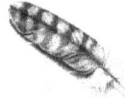

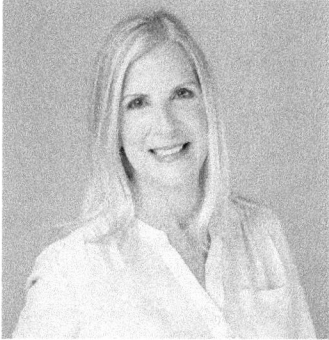

Danni Morford is a wife, and she is also the mother of three sons. Her annual Christmas Letters are written with humor, honesty and raw emotion are about her life as a mom living within the disease of addiction.

Danni's willingness to share her story will help raise awareness about the stigma and shame associated with addiction.

She lives in Austin, Texas, enjoys her time with family and friends, especially at the family ranch.

www.ShootMyAshes.com

Acknowledgments

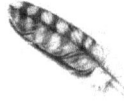

William C. Moyers

~ Author of *Broken: My Story of Redemption and Recovery*

Your book was the first to help me understand addiction and how Travis struggled. Thank you for being authentic, easy to talk with, gracious and giving of your time and support. Your advice to "write a page a day" made this project seem doable. Most of all, thank you for your friendship.

Andrew Wainwright

~ Author of *It's Not Okay to be a Cannibal: How to stop Addiction from Eating your Family Alive*

Thank you for your early interest and continued support. Your advice to use the epistolary style gave me what I needed to bring my book to life. Thank you for believing in me.

Sandy Swenson

~ Author of *The Joey Song and Tending Dandelions*

Thank you for your time, advice, encouragement, and friendship. Your work is an inspiration to me. "No more shame. No more blame."

Hannah Munden, *you were with me from the very beginning of my journey. Your support and encouragement of my writing has meant the world to me.*

Ellie, Gina, and Diane, *you helped me connect with my writing, gave me a safe space to write, and helped me find my voice. Ellie, thank you also for early-stage edits, feedback, and heartfelt support.*

Becky, *thank you for believing in me, and thank you for connecting me with influential literary talents; they believe in me too.*

To all my friends and family, thank you for your love, support and prayers.

Lisa Bovee, *I am so blessed to have you as my editor and one who understands the heart of a mother and the loss of a son. I feel so lucky to have you as a friend as well. You can read my mind and you know what I want to say better than I can say it myself! You made a professional work out of the dreams of an amateur.*

Resources

If you are (or someone you love is) struggling with addiction, help and information are just a click or phone call away:

Hazeldon Betty Ford Foundation
www.HazeldonBettyFord.org
855.668.8506

Al-Anon
www.Al-Anon.org
wso@al-anon.org
888.425.2666

Assistance in Recovery (AiR)
A next-generation behavioral healthcare company
www.aircarehealth.com
800.561.8158

University High School
Safe. Sober. Scholastic.
Austin, Texas
www.UHighSchool.com
info@uhighschool.com
1.512.382.0072

The Christi Center (grief support)
Non-profit org.

www.christicenter.org
512-467-2600
2306 Hancock Drive
Austin, Tx. 78756

Austin Recovery (supportive outpatient
programs)
4201 S Congress Ave #202
Austin, TX 78745
512-697-8635

Alpha/180 (sober co-ed college student
clubhouse)
1-833-257-4218
1904 Nueces
Austin, Tx. 78705
Alpha/180.com

Lisa Bovee Founder of Guided by Grief
Lisa is an author, editor & motivational speaker
www.guidedbygrief.com

Sandy Swenson is the author of The Joey Song and
Tending Dandelions
Her website provides resources, events, books,
CDs and other resources which are helpful for
those living with addiction.
www.sandyswenson.com

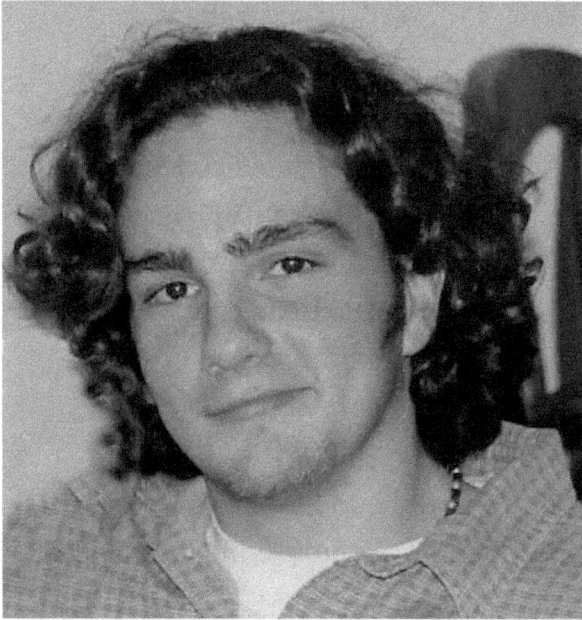

Travis 11.27.1981 - 07.08.2007

Letters of Support

From the desk of Andrew Wainwright
St. Paul, Minnesota

Dear Reader,

There is a story that has been making the rounds of the finer coffee shops and Al-Anon pot lucks of Austin Texas recently. The story goes that a local woman, grief stricken over the loss of her son to the disease of addiction, read a book by a man who lived in Minnesota and reached out him for advice. She told him that in an effort to process her son's loss she had begun to put pen to paper and would he read what she had written? They talked off and on for a few months before life carried them both in different directions. They weren't to speak again for 10 years. Over that time however, a single word from their conversations stayed with her - epistolary. An epistolary story, he had told her, was one told exclusively through letters. She never forgot that word.

In the Fall of 2018, here in St. Paul Minnesota, I was headed into a local restaurant for dinner when I heard my name, "Andrew Wainwright!" shouted in a deep West Texas accent. I looked up to see a woman I had never met before but knew intimately; Mrs. Danni Fourton Morford. Though a decade had passed since we had spoken on the phone, I recognized her instantly. Like survivors of a plane crash, we were intimately bound together in the places where we had individually healed ourselves. I smiled and hugged her deeply.

In our brief exchange that evening two things occurred. First, she told me that her book was complete. Second, she told me that she had made it a book of letters, an epistolary story. As she explained it, that one word had carried her forward through the years as she pursued the tasks that, even in her grief, she remained responsible for: raising two other sons, a marriage, a family, loving, work, play, catharsis, and the timeless and endless pursuit of grace.

I say responsible because we all make choices at the various crossroads of our lives. Danni's choice to live, in the face of losing a child, becomes clear in the pages that follow as she carries forward in time, both on foot and by pen. She abides.

Danni had completed her book. She now set me a task. "Write me a letter to introduce my letters," she said. "With joy and gratitude," I replied.

I have no idea if Danni ever wrote a single letter in her life before she wrote the first Christmas letter in 2004 but God enters through the wound. When she let me read it, I recognized the voice. Heartbroken? Certainly. Honest and funny?

Absolutely. But, more than anything, it was the voice of someone capable of standing poised and reflective at the windblown crossroads of addiction and recovery. Someone who was a true believer in the possibility of possibility. Someone willing to put their grief in service to the greater good.

There is little for me to say other than that the wonder and joy that I first felt upon reading the earliest Christmas Letters so many years ago returned to me when I read this full gathering that lies on the pages beyond.

This is an experiential book about human hearts, spiritual transformation, families, secrets, wonder, and craziness. It is a celebration. It is a book of medicine.

And so, we abide.

From Sandra Swenson
Author, Advocate
Sandysweson.com
Mompower.org

There's no underestimating the power of moms connecting with other moms, maybe especially when a child has been stolen away by the disease of addiction. The more honest and open, the deeper the connection of hearts – so with her collection of raw and intimate letters, Danni is sure to bring a world of help and healing to hurting moms.

With Shoot My Ashes from a Cannon: Beyond Addiction – The Letters, Danni gently pulls us into the reality of her world, day by day, letter by letter, capturing the innermost thoughts and feelings of mothers with addicted children. Haunting and hopeful, full of love and grief, laughs, chills and tears, her book will touch the hearts of mothers on the same journey, as well as open eyes, hearts and minds to the hidden truths of the disease of addiction.

Exquisitely painful and achingly gorgeous, Danni's collection of letters is a true gift.